MW01594845

YOUR GUIDE TO
Healthy Sleep

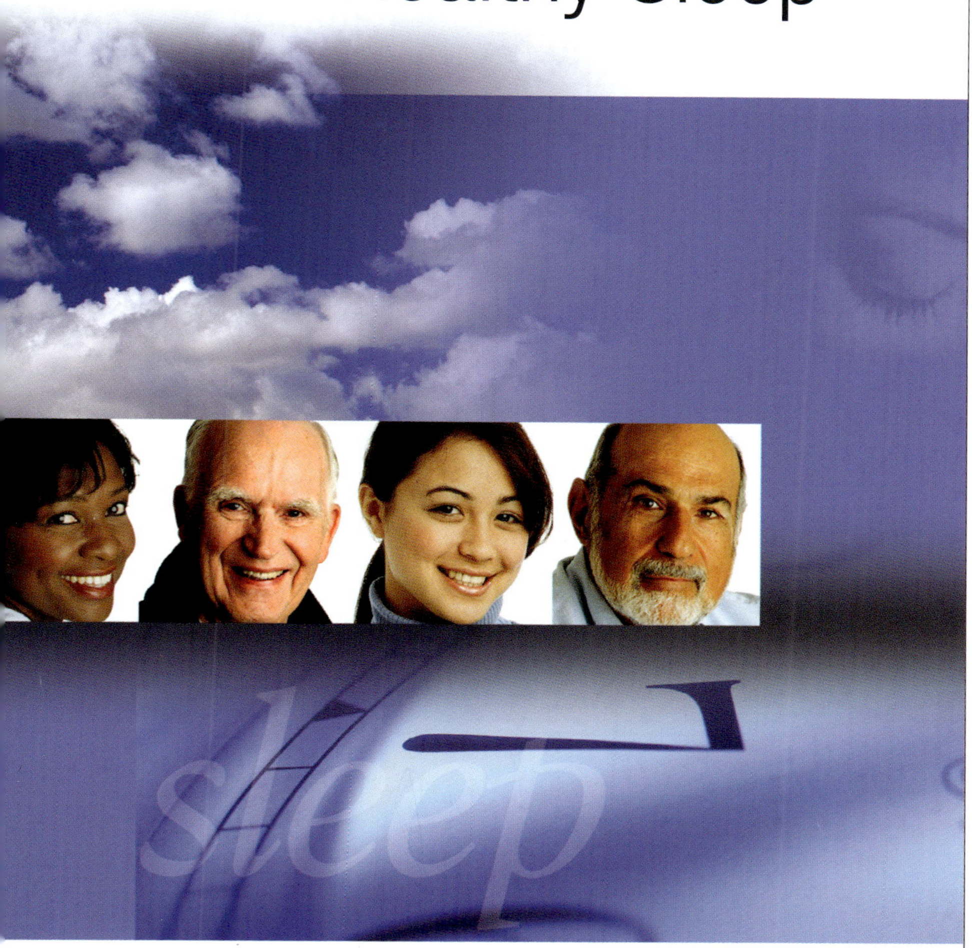

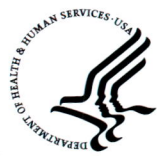

U.S. DEPARTMENT OF HEALTH AND HUMAN SERVICES
National Institutes of Health
National Heart, Lung, and Blood Institute

NIH Publication No. 06-5271
November 2005

Written by: Margie Patlak

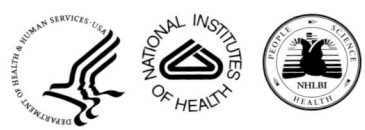

U.S. DEPARTMENT OF HEALTH AND HUMAN SERVICES
National Institutes of Health
National Heart, Lung, and Blood Institute

Contents

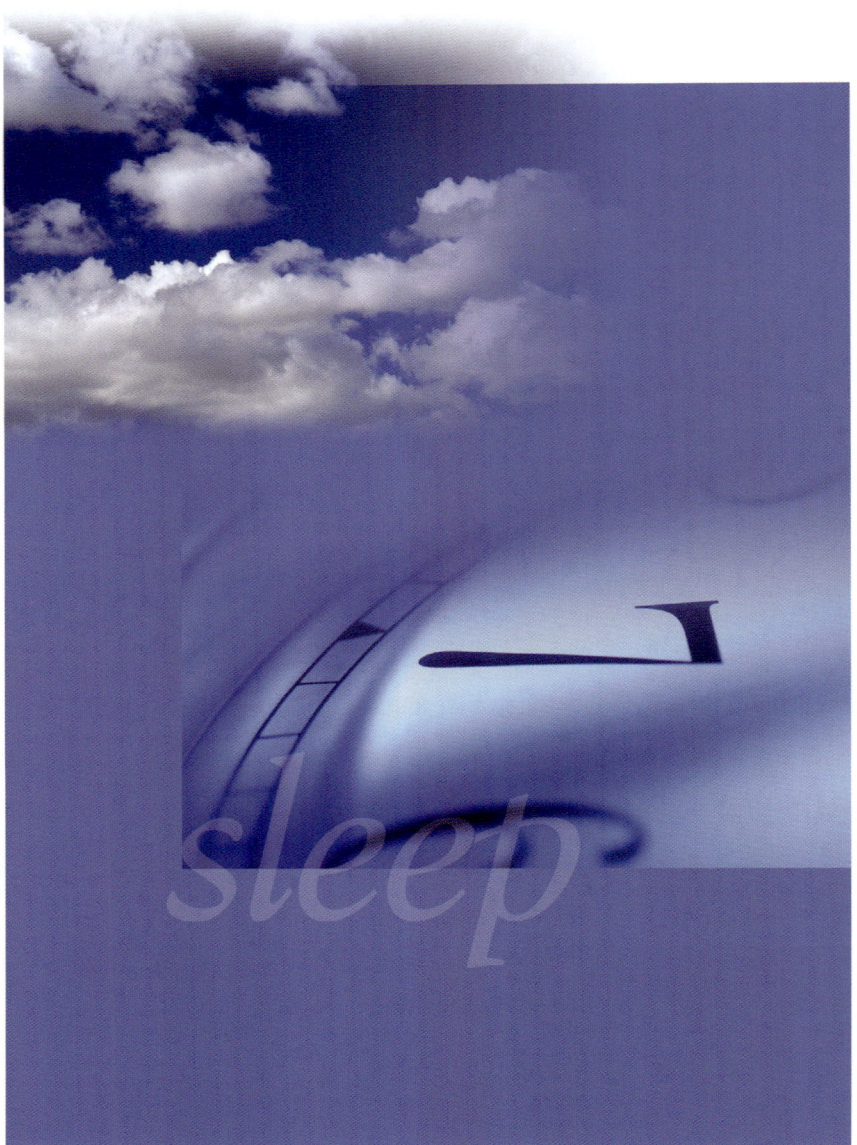

sleep

Introduction

Think of everything you do during your day. Try to guess which activity is so important you should devote one-third of your time to doing it. Probably the first things that come to mind are working, spending time with your family, or pursuing leisure activities. But there's something else you should be doing about one-third of your time—sleeping.

Many people view sleep as merely a "down time" when their brain shuts off and their body rests. In a rush to meet work, school, family, or household responsibilities, people cut back on their sleep, thinking it won't be a problem, because all of these other activities seem much more important. But research reveals that a number of vital tasks carried out during sleep help to maintain good health and enable people to function at their best.

While you sleep, your brain is hard at work forming the pathways necessary for learning and creating memories and new insights. Without enough sleep, you can't focus and pay attention or respond quickly. A lack of sleep may even cause mood problems. In addition, growing evidence shows that a chronic lack of sleep increases the risk for developing obesity, diabetes, cardiovascular disease, and infections.

Despite the mounting support for the notion that adequate sleep, like adequate nutrition and physical activity, is vital to our well-being, people are sleeping less. The nonstop "24/7" nature of the world today encourages longer or nighttime work hours and offers continual access to entertainment and other activities. To keep up, people cut back on sleep. A common myth is that people can learn to get by on little sleep (such as *less than 6 hours* a night) with no adverse consequences. Research suggests, however, that adults need at least 7–8 hours of sleep each night to be well rested. Indeed, in 1910, most people slept 9 hours a night. But recent surveys show the average adult now sleeps *less than 7 hours* a night, and more than one-third of adults report daytime sleepiness so severe that it interferes with work and social functioning at least a few days each month. As many as 70 million Americans may be affected by chronic sleep loss or sleep disorders, at an annual cost of $16 billion in health care expenses and $50 billion in lost productivity.

What happens when you don't get enough sleep? Can you make up for lost sleep during the week by sleeping more on the weekends? How does sleep change as you become older? Is snoring a problem? How can you tell if you have a sleep disorder? Read on to find the answers to these questions and to better understand what sleep is and why it is so necessary. Learn about common sleep myths and practical tips for getting adequate sleep, coping with jet lag and nighttime shift work, and avoiding dangerous drowsy driving. Many common sleep disorders go unrecognized and thus are not treated. This booklet also gives the latest information on sleep disorders such as insomnia, sleep apnea, restless legs syndrome, narcolepsy, and parasomnias.

"When I think of every step in my life, sleep, or lack of sleep, was really instrumental in speeding me up or slowing me down, respectively."

Vice Admiral Richard H. Carmona, M.D., M.P.H., F.A.C.S., U.S. Surgeon General, made these remarks at the 2004 National Sleep Conference at the National Institutes of Health. See conference results and remarks at http://www.nhlbi.nih.gov/meetings/slp_front.htm.

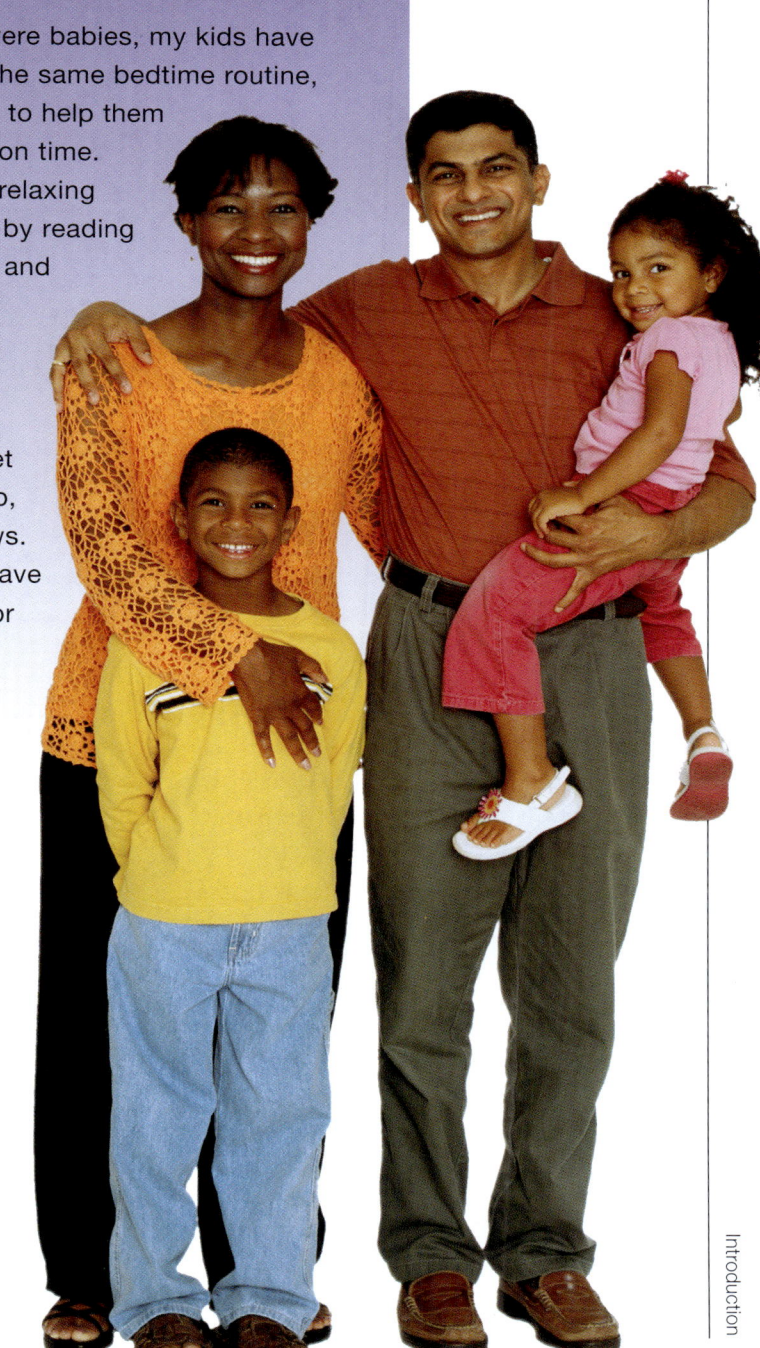

JEANETTE GUYTON-KRISHNAN AND FAMILY

"Since they were babies, my kids have always had the same bedtime routine, and it seems to help them get to sleep on time. We create a relaxing environment by reading them stories and rubbing their backs before they go to sleep. If the kids don't get enough sleep, it really shows. They don't have the energy for school or playing."

What Is Sleep?

Sleep was long considered just a uniform block of time when you are not awake. Thanks to sleep studies done over the past several decades, it is now known that sleep has distinct stages that cycle throughout the night in predictable patterns. How well rested you are and how well you function depend not just on your total sleep time but on how much of the various stages of sleep you get each night.

Your brain stays active throughout sleep, and each stage of sleep is linked to a distinctive pattern of electrical activity known as brain waves.

Sleep is divided into two basic types: rapid eye movement (REM) sleep and non-REM sleep (with four different stages). (See "Types of Sleep" on page 5.) Typically, sleep begins with non-REM sleep. In stage 1 non-REM sleep, you sleep lightly and can be awakened easily by noises or other disturbances. During this first stage of sleep, your eyes move slowly, and your muscle activity slows. You then enter stage 2 non-REM sleep, when your eye movements stop. Your brain shows a distinctive pattern of slower brain waves with occasional bursts of rapid waves.

When you progress into stage 3 non-REM sleep, your brain waves become even slower, although they are still punctuated by smaller, faster waves. By stage 4 non-REM sleep, the brain produces extremely slow waves almost exclusively. Stages 3 and 4 are considered deep sleep, during which it is very difficult to be awakened. Children who wet the bed or sleep walk tend to do so during stages 3 or 4 of non-REM sleep. Deep sleep is considered the "restorative" part of sleep that is necessary for feeling well rested and energetic during the day.

During REM sleep, your eyes move rapidly in various directions, even though your eyelids remain closed. Your breathing also becomes more rapid, irregular, and shallow, and your heart rate and

Types of
Sleep

Non-REM Sleep		REM Sleep
Stage 1:	Light sleep; easily awakened; muscle activity; eye movements slow down.	Usually first occurs about 90 minutes after you fall asleep; cycles along with the non-REM stages throughout the night. Eyes move rapidly, with eyelids closed. Breathing is more rapid, irregular, and shallow. Heart rate and blood pressure increase. Dreaming occurs. Arm and leg muscles are temporarily paralyzed.
Stage 2:	Eye movements stop; slower brain waves, with occasional bursts of rapid brain waves.	
Stage 3:	Considered deep sleep; difficult to awaken; brain waves slow down more, but still have occasional rapid waves.	
Stage 4:	Considered deep sleep; difficult to awaken; extremely slow brain waves.	

Types of Sleep

blood pressure increase. Dreaming typically occurs during REM sleep. During this type of sleep, your arm and leg muscles are temporarily paralyzed so that you cannot "act out" any dreams that you may be having.

The first period of REM sleep you experience usually occurs about an hour to an hour and a half after falling asleep. After that, the sleep stages repeat themselves continuously while you sleep. As the night progresses, REM sleep time becomes longer, while time spent in non-REM sleep stages 3 and 4 becomes shorter. By morning, nearly all your sleep time is spent in stages 1 and 2 of non-REM sleep and in REM sleep. If REM sleep is disrupted during one night, REM sleep time is typically longer than normal in subsequent nights until you catch up. Overall, almost one-half your total sleep time is spent in stages 1 and 2 non-REM sleep and about one-fifth each in deep sleep (stages 3 and 4 of non-REM sleep) and REM sleep. In contrast, infants spend half or more of their total sleep time in REM sleep. Gradually, as they mature, the percentage of total sleep time they spend in REM progressively decreases to reach the one-fifth level typical of later childhood and adulthood.

Why people dream and why REM sleep is so important are not well understood. It is known that REM sleep stimulates the brain regions used in learning and the laying down of memories. Animal studies suggest that dreams may reflect the brain's sorting and selectively storing important new information acquired during wake time. While this information is processed, the brain might revisit scenes from the day while pulling up older memories. This process may explain why childhood memories can be interspersed with more recent events during dreams. Studies show, however, that other stages of sleep besides REM are also needed to form the pathways in the brain that enable us to learn and remember.

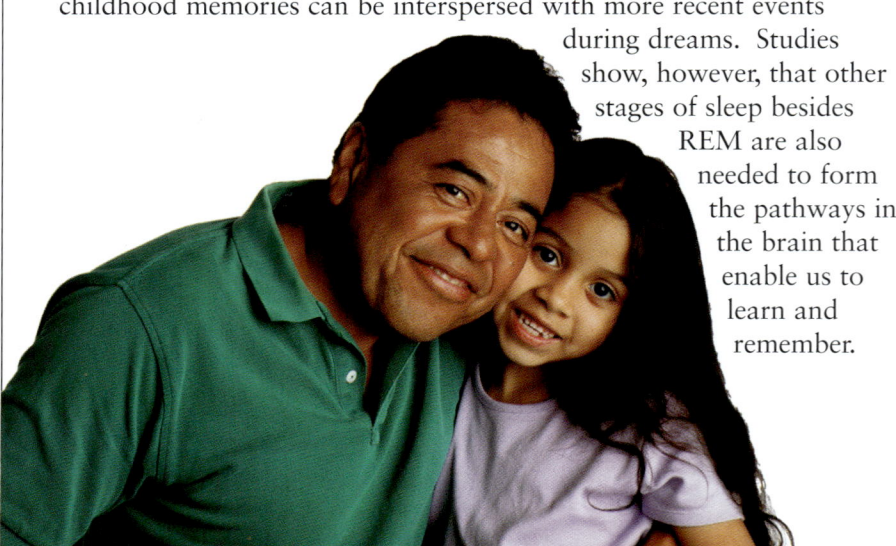

What Makes You Sleep?

Although you may put off going to sleep in order to squeeze more activities into your day, eventually your need for sleep becomes overwhelming and you are forced to get some sleep. This daily drive for sleep appears to be due, in part, to a compound known as adenosine. This natural chemical builds up in your blood as time awake increases. While you sleep, your body breaks down the adenosine. Thus, this molecule may be what your body uses to keep track of lost sleep and to trigger sleep when needed. An accumulation of adenosine and other factors might explain why, after several nights of less than optimal amounts of sleep, you build up a sleep debt that you must make up by sleeping longer than normal. Because of such built-in molecular feedback, you can't adapt to getting less sleep than your body needs. Eventually, a lack of sleep catches up with you.

The time of day when you feel sleepy and go to sleep is also governed by your internal "biological clock" and environmental cues—the most important being light and darkness. Your biological clock is actually a tiny bundle of cells in your brain that responds to light signals received through your eyes. When darkness falls, the biological clock triggers the production of the hormone melatonin. This hormone makes you feel drowsy as it continues to increase during the night. Because of your biological clock, you naturally feel the most sleepy between midnight and 7 a.m. You may also feel a second and milder daily "low" in the midafternoon between 1 p.m. and 4 p.m. At that time, another rise occurs in melatonin production and might make you feel sleepy.

Your biological clock makes you the most alert during daylight hours and the most drowsy in the early morning hours. Consequently, most people do their best work during the day. Our 24/7 society, however, demands that some people work at night. Nearly one-quarter of all workers work shifts that are not during the daytime, and more than two-thirds of these workers have problem sleepiness and/or difficulty sleeping. Because their work schedules are at odds with powerful sleep-regulating cues like sunlight, night shift workers often find themselves drowsy at work, and they have difficulty falling or staying asleep during the daylight hours when their work schedules require them to sleep.

The fatigue experienced by night shift workers can be dangerous. Major industrial accidents—such as the Three Mile Island and Chernobyl nuclear power plant accidents and the Exxon Valdez oil spill—have been caused, in part, by mistakes made by overly tired workers on the night shift or an extended shift.

Night shift workers also are at greater risk of being in car crashes when they drive home from work. One study found that one-fifth of night shift workers had a car crash or a near miss in the preceding year because of sleepiness on the drive home from work. Night shift workers are also more likely to have physical problems, such as heart disease, digestive disturbances, and infertility, as well as emotional problems. All of these problems may be related, at least in part, to the workers' chronic sleepiness. See "Working the Night Shift" on page 9 for some helpful tips.

Other factors can also influence your need for sleep, including your immune system's production of cellular hormones called cytokines. These compounds are made in large quantities in response to certain infectious diseases or chronic inflammation and may prompt you to sleep more than usual. The extra sleep may help you conserve the resources needed to fight the infection. Recent studies confirm that being well rested improves the body's responses to infection.

People are creatures of habit, and one of the hardest habits to break is the natural wake and sleep cycle. A number of physiological factors conspire to help you sleep and wake up at the same times each day. Consequently, you may have a hard time adjusting when you travel across time zones. The light cues outside and the clocks in your new location may tell you it is 8 a.m. and you should be active, but your body is telling you it is more like 4 a.m. and you should sleep. The end result is jet lag—sleepiness during the day, difficulty falling or staying asleep at night, poor concentration, confusion, nausea, and general malaise and irritability. See "Dealing With Jet Lag" on page 10.

Working the
Night Shift

Try to limit night shift work, if that is possible. If you must work the night shift, the following tips may help you:

- Increase your total amount of sleep by adding naps and lengthening the amount of time you allot for sleep.
- Use bright lights in your workplace.
- Minimize your shift changes so that your body's biological clock can adjust to a nighttime work schedule.
- Get rid of sound and light distractions in your bedroom during your daytime sleep.
- Use caffeine only during the first part of your shift to promote alertness at night.

If you are unable to fall asleep during the day, and all else fails, talk with your doctor to see if it would be wise for you to use prescribed, short-acting sleeping pills to help you sleep during the day.

Night Shift

Dealing With
Jet Lag

Eastward travel generally causes more severe jet lag than westward travel because traveling east requires you to shorten the day, and your biological clock is better able to adjust to a longer day than a shorter day. Fortunately for globetrotters, a few preventive measures and treatments seem to help some people relieve jet lag:

- **Adjust your biological clock.** Several days before traveling to a new time zone, gradually shift your sleeping and eating times to coincide with those at your destination. You can also adjust your clock by using light therapy. This involves being exposed to special lights, many times brighter than ordinary household light, for several hours near the time you want to wake up. Alternatively, after arrival, spend a lot of time outdoors to make sure your body gets the light cues it needs to adjust to the new time zone.

- **Avoid alcohol and caffeine.** Although it may be tempting to drink alcohol to relieve the stress of travel and make it easier to fall asleep, you're more likely to sleep lighter and wake up in the middle of the night when the effects of the alcohol wear off. Caffeine can help keep you awake longer, but caffeine can also make it harder for you to fall asleep if its effects haven't worn off by the time you are ready to go to bed.

- **What about melatonin?** Your body produces this hormone that makes you drowsy. Melatonin builds up in your body as the night progresses and decreases when daylight arrives.

Melatonin is available as an over-the-counter supplement. Because melatonin is considered safe when used over a period of days or weeks and seems to contribute to feeling sleepy, it has been suggested as a treatment for jet lag. But melatonin's effectiveness is controversial, and its safety when used over a prolonged period is unclear. Some studies find that taking melatonin supplements before bedtime for several days after arrival in a new time zone can make it easier to fall asleep at the proper time. Other studies find that melatonin does not help to relieve jet lag.

Be aware that adjusting to a new time zone may take several days. If you are going to be away for just a few days, it may be better to stick to your original sleep and wake times as much as possible, rather than adjusting your biological clock too many times in rapid succession.

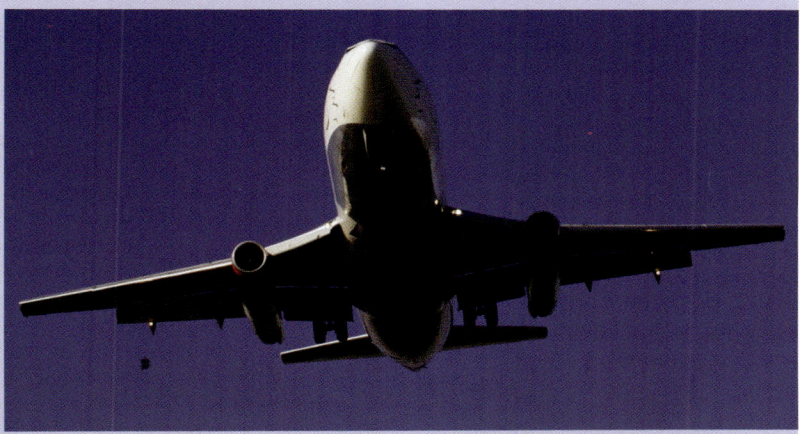

Jet Lag

What Does Sleep Do for You?

A number of tasks vital to health and quality of life are linked to sleep, and these tasks are impaired when you are sleep deprived.

Learning, Memory, and Mood

Students who have trouble grasping new information or learning new skills are often advised to "sleep on it," and that advice seems well founded. Recent studies reveal that people can learn a task better if they are well rested. They also can remember better what they learned if they get a good night's sleep after learning the task than if they are sleep deprived. Volunteers had to sleep at least 6 hours to show improvement in learning, and the amount of improvement was directly tied to how much time they slept. In other words, volunteers who slept 8 hours outperformed those who slept only 6 or 7 hours. Other studies suggest that all the benefits of training for mentally challenging tasks are maximized after a good night's sleep, rather than immediately following the training or after sleeping for a short period overnight.

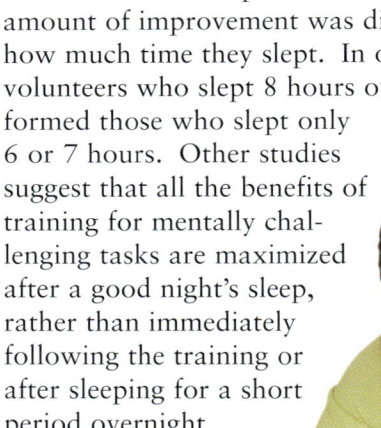

Many well-known artists and scientists claim to have had creative insights while they slept. Mary Shelley, for example, said

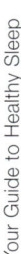

the idea for her novel *Frankenstein* came to her in a dream. Although it has not been shown that dreaming is the driving force behind innovation, one study suggests that sleep is needed for creative problem solving. In that study, volunteers were asked to perform a memory task and then were tested 8 hours later. Those who were allowed to sleep for 8 hours immediately after receiving the task and before being tested were much more likely to find a creative way of simplifying the task and improving their performance compared to those who were awake the entire 8 hours before being tested.

Exactly what happens during sleep to improve our learning, memory, and insight isn't known. Experts suspect, however, that while people sleep, they form or reinforce the pathways of brain cells needed to perform these tasks. This process may explain why sleep is needed for proper brain development in infants.

Not only is a good night's sleep required to form new learning and memory pathways in the brain, but sleep is also necessary for those pathways to work up to speed. Several studies show that lack of sleep causes thinking processes to slow down. Lack of sleep also makes it harder to focus and pay attention. Lack of sleep can make you more easily confused. Studies also find a lack of sleep leads to faulty decisionmaking and more risk taking. A lack of sleep slows down your reaction time, which is particularly significant to driving and other tasks that require quick response. When people who lack sleep are tested by using a driving simulator, they perform just as poorly as people who are drunk. (See "Crash in Bed Not on the Road" on page 16.) The bottom line is: not getting a good night's sleep can be dangerous!

Even if you don't have a mentally or physically challenging day ahead of you, you should still get enough sleep to put yourself in a good mood. Most people report being irritable, if not downright unhappy, when they lack sleep. People who chronically suffer from a lack of sleep, either because they do not spend enough time in bed or because they have an untreated sleep disorder, are at greater risk of developing depression. One group of people who usually don't get enough sleep is mothers of newborns. Some experts think depression after childbirth (postpartum blues) is caused, in part, by a lack of sleep.

Your Heart

Sleep gives your heart and vascular system a much-needed rest. During non-REM sleep, your heart rate and blood pressure progressively slow as you enter deeper sleep. During REM sleep, your heart rate and blood pressure have boosted spikes of activity. Overall, however, sleep reduces your heart rate and blood pressure by about 10 percent.

If you don't get enough sleep, this nightly dip in blood pressure, which appears to be important for good cardiovascular health, may not occur. According to several studies, if your blood pressure does not dip during sleep, you are more likely to experience strokes, chest pain known as angina, an irregular heartbeat, and heart attacks. You are also more likely to develop congestive heart failure, a condition in which fluid builds up in the body because the heart is not pumping sufficiently. Failure to experience the normal dip in blood pressure during sleep can be related to insufficient sleep time, an untreated sleep disorder, or other factors. African Americans, for example, tend not to have as much of a dip in blood pressure during sleep. This difference may help to explain why they are more likely than Caucasians to have serious cardiovascular disease.

A lack of sleep also puts your body under stress and may trigger the release of more adrenaline, cortisol, and other stress hormones during the day. These hormones contribute to your blood pressure not dipping during sleep, thereby increasing the risk for heart disease. Inadequate sleep may also negatively affect your heart and vascular system by the increased production of certain proteins thought to play a role in heart disease. For example, some studies find that people who chronically do not get enough sleep have higher blood levels of C-reactive protein. Higher levels of this protein may suggest a greater risk of developing hardening of the arteries (atherosclerosis).

Your Hormones

When you were young, your mother may have told you that you need to get enough sleep to grow strong and tall. She may have been right! Deep sleep triggers more release of growth hormone, which fuels growth in children and boosts muscle mass and the repair of cells and tissues in children and adults. Sleep's effect on the release of sex hormones also encourages puberty and fertility.

Consequently, women who work at night and tend to lack sleep are, therefore, more likely to have trouble conceiving or to miscarry.

Your mother also probably was right if she told you that getting a good night's sleep on a regular basis would help keep you from getting sick and help you get better if you do get sick. During sleep, your body creates more cytokines—cellular hormones that help the immune system fight various infections. Lack of sleep can reduce the ability to fight off common infections. Research also reveals that a lack of sleep can reduce the body's response to the flu vaccine. For example, sleep-deprived volunteers given the flu vaccine produced less than half as many flu antibodies as those who were well rested and given the same vaccine.

Although lack of exercise and other factors are important contributors, the current epidemic of diabetes and obesity appears to be related, at least in part, to chronically getting inadequate sleep. Evidence is growing that sleep is a powerful regulator of appetite, energy use, and weight control. During sleep, the body's production of the appetite suppressor *leptin* increases, and the appetite stimulant *grehlin* decreases. Studies find that the less people sleep, the more likely they are to be overweight or obese and prefer eating foods that are higher in calories and carbohydrates. People who report an average total sleep time of 5 hours a night, for example, are much more likely to become obese compared to people who sleep 7–8 hours a night.

A number of hormones released during sleep also control the body's use of energy. A distinct rise and fall of blood sugar levels during sleep appears to be linked to sleep stage. Not getting enough sleep overall or enough of each stage of sleep disrupts this pattern. One study found that, when healthy young men slept only 4 hours a night for 6 nights in a row, their insulin and blood sugar levels mimicked those seen in people who were developing diabetes. Another study found that women who slept *less than 7 hours* a night were more likely to develop diabetes over time than those who slept between 7 and 8 hours a night.

Crash in Bed
Not on the Road

Most people are aware of the hazards of drunk driving. But driving while sleepy can be just as dangerous. Indeed, crashes due to sleepy drivers are as deadly as those due to drivers impaired by alcohol. And you don't have to be asleep at the wheel to put yourself and others in danger. Both alcohol and a lack of sleep hamper your ability to react quickly to a suddenly braking car, a sharp curve in the road, or other situations that require rapid responses. Just a few seconds' delay in reaction time can be a life-or-death matter when driving. When people who lack sleep are tested by using a driving simulator, they perform as badly or worse than those who are drunk. The combination of alcohol and lack of sleep can be especially dangerous.

Of course, driving is also hazardous if you fall asleep at the wheel, which happens surprisingly often. One-quarter of the drivers surveyed in New York State reported they had fallen asleep at the wheel at some time. Often, people briefly nod off at the wheel without being aware of it—they just can't recall what happened over the previous few seconds or longer. And people who lack sleep are more apt to take risks and make poor judgments, which can also boost their chances of getting in a car crash.

Here are some potentially life-saving tips for avoiding drowsy driving:

- **Be well rested before hitting the road.** If you have several nights in a row of fewer than 7–8 hours of sleep, your reaction time slows. Restoring that reaction time to normal often takes more than 1 night of good sleep, because your sleep debt accumulates after each night you lose sleep. It may take several nights of being well rested to repay that sleep debt and ensure that you are ready for driving on a long road trip.

- **Avoid driving between midnight and 7 a.m.** Unless you are accustomed to being awake then, this period of time is when we are naturally the most tired.
- **Don't drive alone.** A companion who can keep you engaged in conversation might help you stay awake while driving.
- **Schedule frequent breaks on long road trips.** If you feel sleepy while driving, pull off the road and take a nap for 15–20 minutes.
- **Don't drink alcohol.** Just one beer when you are sleep deprived will affect you as much as two or three beers when you are well rested.
- **Don't count on caffeine.** Although drinking a cola or a cup of coffee might help keep you awake for a short time, it won't overcome excessive sleepiness or relieve a sleep debt.

Opening a window or turning up the radio won't help you stay awake while driving. Be aware of these warning signs that you are too sleepy to drive safely: trouble keeping your eyes focused, continual yawning, or being unable to recall driving the last few miles. Remember, if you are short on sleep, stay out of the driver's seat!

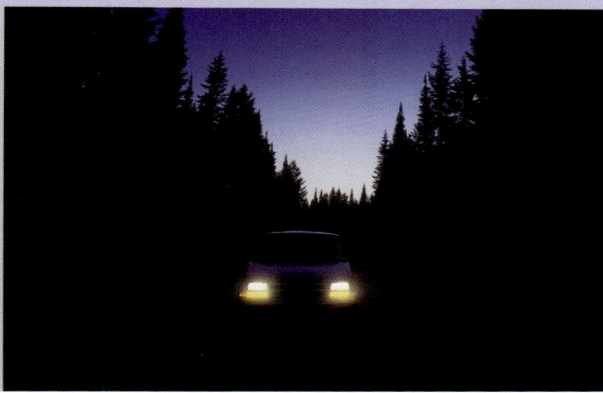

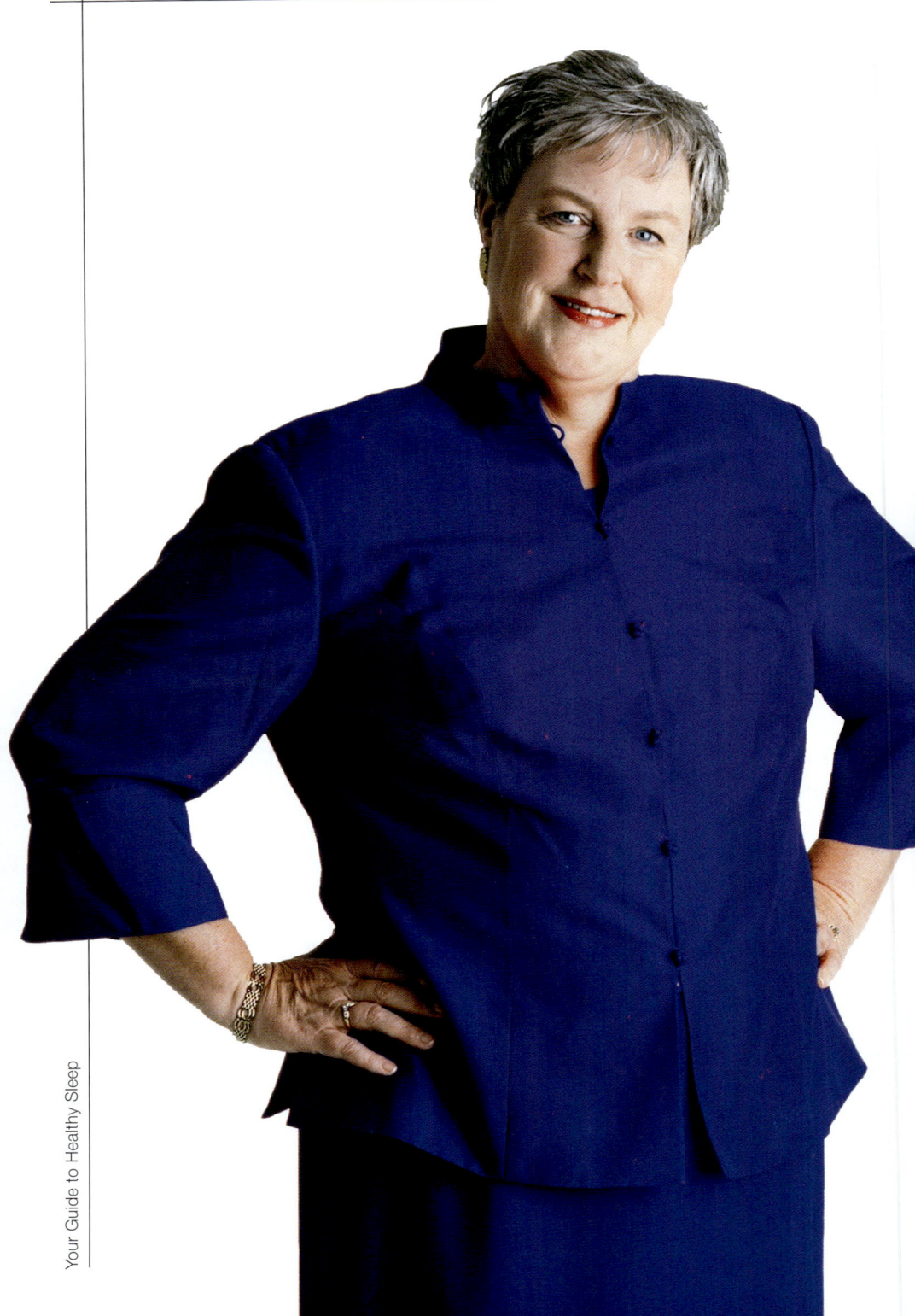

How Much Sleep Is Enough?

Animal studies suggest that sleep is as vital as food for survival. Rats, for example, normally live 2–3 years, but they live only 5 weeks if they are deprived of REM sleep and only 2–3 weeks if they are deprived of all sleep stages—a timeframe similar to death due to starvation. But how much sleep do humans need? To help answer that question, scientists look at how much people sleep when unrestricted, the average amount of sleep among various age groups, and the amount of sleep that studies reveal is necessary to function at your best.

When healthy adults are given unlimited opportunity to sleep, they sleep on average between 8 and 8.5 hours a night. But sleep needs vary from person to person. Some people appear to need only about 7 hours to avoid problem sleepiness whereas others need 9 or more hours of sleep. Sleep needs also change throughout the lifecycle. Newborns sleep between 16 and 18 hours a day, and children in preschool sleep between 10 and 12 hours a day. School-aged children and adolescents need at least 9 hours of sleep a night.

The hormonal influences of puberty tend to shift adolescents' biological clocks. As a result, teenagers are more likely to go to bed later than younger children and adults, and they tend to want to sleep later in the morning. This sleep–wake rhythm is contrary to the early-morning start times of many high schools and helps explain why most teenagers get an average of only 7–7.5 hours of sleep a night.

As people get older, the pattern of sleep also changes—especially the amount of time spent in the deep sleep stages. Children spend more time than adults in these sleep stages. This explains why children can sleep through loud noises and why they might not wake up when they are moved from the car to their beds. During adolescence, a big drop occurs in the amount of time spent in deep sleep, which is replaced by lighter, stage 2 sleep. Between young adulthood and midlife, the percentage of deep sleep falls again—from less than 20 percent to less than 5 percent, one study suggests—and is replaced with lighter sleep (stages 1 and 2). From midlife through late life, people's sleep has more interruptions by wakefulness during the night. This disruption causes older persons to lose more and more of stages 1 and 2 non-REM sleep as well as REM sleep.

Many older people complain of difficulty falling asleep, early morning awakenings, frequent and long awakenings during the night, daytime sleepiness, and a lack of refreshing sleep. Many sleep problems, however, are not a natural aspect of sleep in the elderly. Because older people are more likely to have many illnesses that can disrupt sleep, their sleep complaints often may be due, in part, to illnesses or the medications used to treat them. In fact, one study found that the prevalence of sleep problems is very low in *healthy* older adults. Other causes of some of older adults' sleep complaints are sleep apnea, restless legs syndrome, and other sleep disorders that become more common with age. Also, older people are more likely to have their sleep disrupted by the need to urinate during the night.

Some evidence shows that the biological clock shifts in older people, so they are more apt to go to sleep earlier at night and wake up earlier in the morning. No evidence indicates that older people can get by with less sleep than younger people. (See "Top 10 Sleep Myths" on page 22.) Poor sleep in older

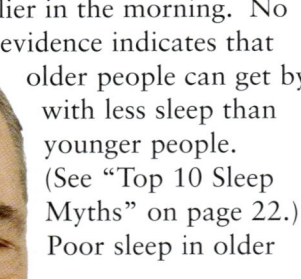

people is linked to excessive daytime sleepiness, attention and memory problems, depressed mood, and overuse of sleeping pills.

Despite variations in sleep quantity and quality, both related to age and between individuals, studies suggest that the optimal amount of sleep needed to perform adequately, avoid a sleep debt, and not have problem sleepiness during the day is about 7–8 hours for adults and 9 or more hours for school-aged children and adolescents. Similar amounts seem to be necessary to avoid further increasing the risk of developing obesity, diabetes, or cardiovascular disorders.

Quality of sleep is as important as quantity. People whose sleep is frequently interrupted or cut short may not get enough of both non-REM sleep and REM sleep. Both types of sleep appear to be crucial for learning and memory—and perhaps for all the other restorative benefits of healthy sleep, including the growth and repair of cells.

Many people try to make up for lost sleep during the week by sleeping more on the weekends. But if you have lost too much sleep, sleeping in on the weekend does not completely erase your sleep debt. Certainly, sleeping more at the end of the week does not make up for the hampered performance you most likely had at the beginning of or during that week. Just 1 night of inadequate sleep can adversely affect your functioning and mood during at least the next day.

Daytime naps are another strategy some people use to make up for lost sleep during the night. Some evidence shows that short naps (up to an hour) can make up, at least partially, for the sleep missed on the previous night and improve alertness, mood, and work performance. But naps don't substitute for a good night's sleep. One study found that a daytime nap after a lack of sleep at night did not fully restore levels of blood sugar to the pattern seen with adequate nighttime sleep. If a nap lasts longer than 1 hour, you may have a hard time waking up fully. In addition, late afternoon naps can make falling asleep at night more difficult.

Top 10
Sleep Myths

Myth 1: Sleep is a time when your body and brain shut down for rest and relaxation.
No evidence shows that any major organ (including the brain) or regulatory system in the body shuts down during sleep. Some physiological processes actually become more active while you sleep. For example, secretion of certain hormones is boosted, and activity of the pathways in the brain needed for learning and memory is heightened.

Myth 2: Getting just 1 hour less sleep per night than needed will not have any effect on your daytime functioning.
This lack of sleep may not make you noticeably sleepy during the day. But even slightly less sleep can affect your ability to think properly and respond quickly, and it can compromise your cardiovascular health and energy balance as well as the ability to fight infections, particularly if lack of sleep continues. If you consistently do not get enough sleep, eventually a sleep debt builds up that will make you excessively tired during the day.

Myth 3: Your body adjusts quickly to different sleep schedules.
Your biological clock makes you most alert during the daytime and most drowsy at night. Thus, even if you work the night shift, you will naturally feel sleepy when nighttime comes. Most people can reset their biological clock, but only by appropriately timed cues—and even then, by 1–2 hours per day at best. Consequently, it can take more than a week to adjust to a dramatically altered sleep/wake cycle, such as you encounter when traveling across several time zones or switching from working the day shift to the night shift.

Sleep Myths

Myth 4: People need less sleep as they get older.

Older people don't need less sleep, but they often *get* less sleep or find their sleep less refreshing. That's because as people age, they spend less time in the deep, restful stages of sleep and are more easily awakened. Older people are also more likely to have insomnia or other medical conditions that disrupt their sleep.

Myth 5: Extra sleep at night can cure you of problems with excessive daytime fatigue.

Not only is the quantity of sleep important but also the *quality* of sleep. Some people sleep 8 or 9 hours a night but don't feel well rested when they wake up because the quality of their sleep is poor. A number of sleep disorders and other medical conditions affect the quality of sleep. Sleeping more won't alleviate the daytime sleepiness these disorders or conditions cause. However, many of these disorders or conditions can be treated effectively with changes in behavior or with medical therapies.

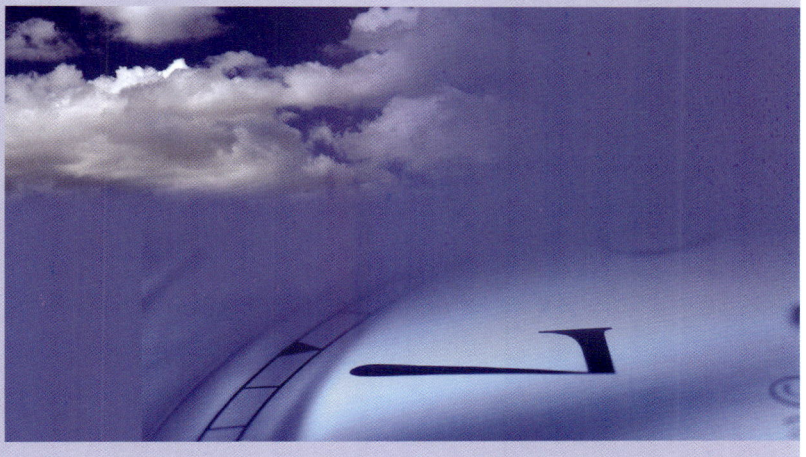

Top 10
Sleep Myths (continued)

Myth 6: You can make up for lost sleep during the week by sleeping more on the weekends.

Although this sleeping pattern will help relieve part of a sleep debt, it will not completely make up for the lack of sleep. This pattern also will not make up for impaired performance during the week because of not sleeping enough. Furthermore, sleeping later on the weekends can affect your biological clock so that it is much harder to go to sleep at the right time on Sunday nights and get up early on Monday mornings.

Myth 7: Naps are a waste of time.

Although naps do not substitute for a good night's sleep, they can be restorative and help counter some of the impaired performance that results from not getting enough sleep at night. Naps can actually help you learn how to do certain tasks quicker. But avoid taking naps later than 3 p.m., as late naps can interfere with your ability to fall asleep at night. Also, limit your naps to no longer than 1 hour because longer naps will make it harder to wake up and get back in the swing of things. If you take frequent naps during the day, you may have a sleep disorder that should be treated.

Myth 8: Snoring is a normal part of sleep.

Snoring during sleep is common, particularly as a person gets older. Evidence is growing that snoring on a regular basis can make you sleepy during the day and more susceptible to diabetes and heart disease. In addition, some studies link frequent snoring to problem behavior and poorer school achievement in children. Loud, frequent snoring can also be a sign of sleep apnea, a serious sleep disorder that should be treated. (See "Is Snoring a Problem?" on page 33.)

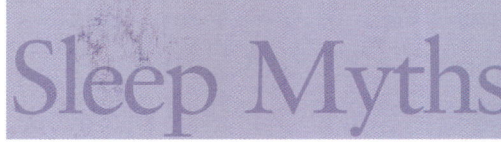

Myth 9: Children who don't get enough sleep at night will show signs of sleepiness during the day.
Unlike adults, children who don't get enough sleep at night typically become more active than normal during the day. They also show difficulty paying attention and behaving properly. Consequently, they may be misdiagnosed as having attention-deficit hyperactivity.

Myth 10: The main cause of insomnia is worry.
Although worry or stress can cause a short bout of insomnia, a persistent inability to fall asleep or stay asleep at night can be caused by a number of other factors. Certain medications and sleep disorders can keep you up at night. Other common causes of insomnia are depression, anxiety disorders, and asthma, arthritis, or other medical conditions with symptoms that become more troublesome at night. Some people who have chronic insomnia also appear to be more revved up than normal, so it is harder for them to fall asleep.

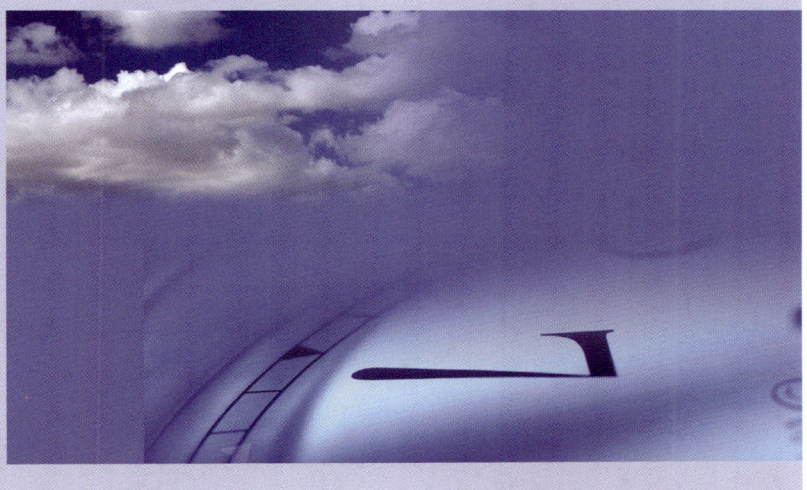

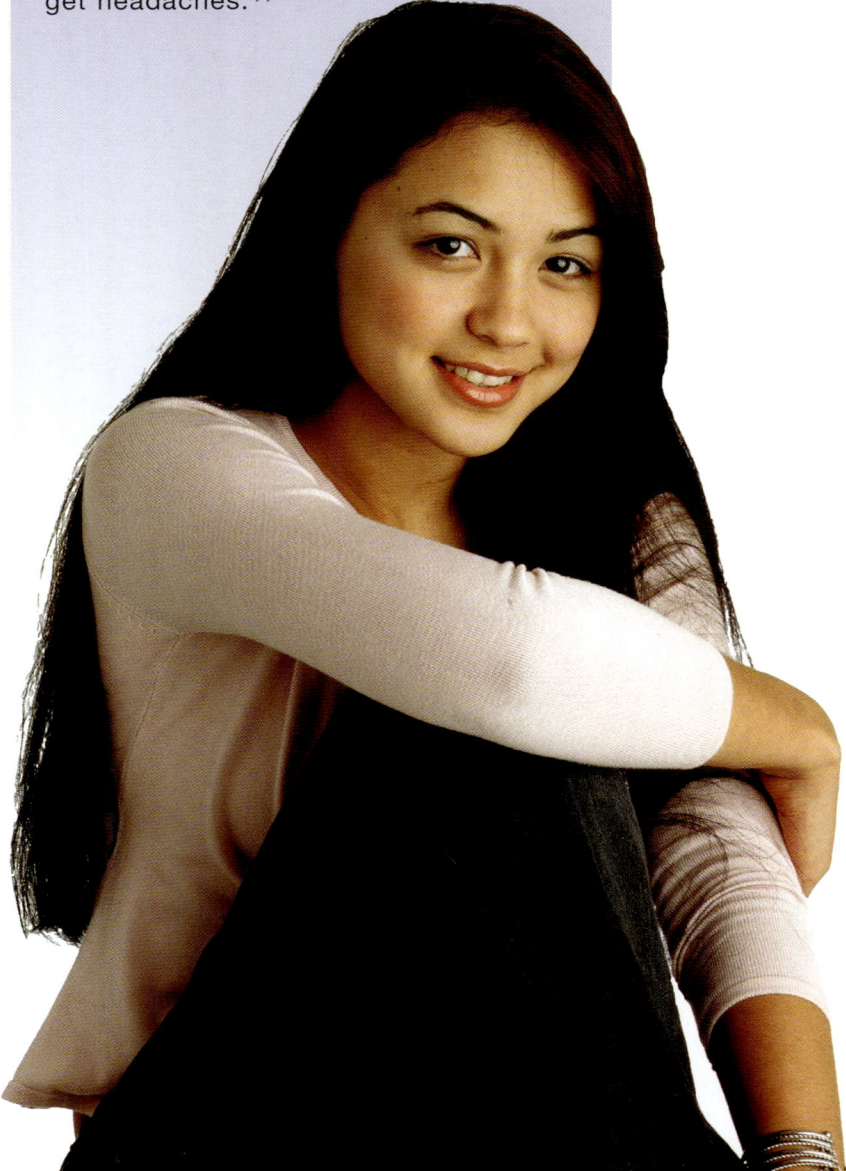

DAPHNE LONDON

" I wake up early to get ready for school. I am tired in the morning and by the end of the school day, I am very tired again. An afterschool nap seems to refresh me and help me focus on homework. Without it, I am grumpy and stressed, can't focus, and sometimes get headaches. "

What Disrupts Sleep?

Many factors can prevent a good night's sleep. These factors range from well-known stimulants, such as coffee, to certain pain relievers, decongestants, and other culprits. Many people depend on the caffeine in coffee, soft drinks (for example, colas), or tea to wake them up in the morning or to keep them awake. Caffeine is thought to block the cell receptors that adenosine uses to trigger its sleep-inducing signals. In this way, caffeine fools the body into thinking it isn't tired. It can take as long as 6–8 hours for the effects of caffeine to wear off completely. Drinking a cup of coffee in the late after-noon consequently may prevent your falling asleep at night.

Nicotine is another stimulant that can keep you awake. Nicotine also leads to lighter than normal sleep. Heavy smokers also tend to wake up too early because of nicotine withdrawal. Although alco-hol is a sedative that makes it easier to fall asleep, it prevents deep sleep and REM sleep, allowing only the lighter stages of sleep. People who drink alcohol also tend to wake up in the middle of the night when the effects of an alcoholic "nightcap" wear off.

Certain commonly used prescription and over-the-counter medicines contain ingredients that can keep you awake. These ingredients include decongestants and steroids. Many pain relievers taken by headache sufferers contain caffeine. Heart and blood pressure med-ications known as "beta blockers" can cause difficulty falling asleep and increase the number of awakenings during the night. People who have chronic asthma or bronchitis also have more problems falling asleep and staying asleep than healthy people, either because of their breathing difficulties or because of the medicines they take. Other chronic painful or uncomfortable conditions—such as arthritis, congestive heart failure, and sickle cell anemia—can disrupt sleep, too.

A number of psychological disorders—including schizophrenia, bipolar disorder, and anxiety disorders—are well known for disrupting sleep. Depression often leads to insomnia, and insomnia can cause depression. Some of these psychological disorders are more likely to disrupt REM sleep. Psychological stress also takes its toll on sleep, making it more difficult to fall asleep or stay asleep. People who feel stressed also tend to spend less time in deep sleep and REM sleep. Many people report having difficulties sleeping if, for example, they have recently lost a loved one, are undergoing a divorce, or are under stress at work.

Menstrual cycle hormones can affect how well women sleep. Progesterone is known to induce sleep and circulates in greater concentrations in the second half of the menstrual cycle. For this reason, women may sleep better during this phase of their menstrual cycle, but many women report trouble sleeping the night before their menstrual bleeding starts. This sleep disruption is probably related to the abrupt drop in progesterone levels in their bodies just before they begin to bleed. Women in their late forties and early fifties, however, report more difficulties sleeping (insomnia) than younger women. These difficulties may be because, as they near or enter menopause, they have lower concentrations of progesterone. Hot flashes in women of this age also may cause sleep disruption and difficulties.

Certain lifestyle factors may also deprive a person of needed sleep. Large meals or exercise just before bedtime can make it harder to fall asleep. Studies show that exercise in the evening delays the extra release of melatonin at night that helps the body fall asleep. Exercise in the daytime, on the other hand, is linked to improved nighttime sleep.

If you aren't getting enough sleep or aren't falling asleep early enough, you may be overscheduling activities that can prevent you from getting the quiet relaxation time you need to prepare for sleep. Most people report that it's easier to fall asleep if they have time to wind down into a less active state before sleeping. Relaxing in a hot bath before bedtime may help. In addition, your body temperature drops after a hot bath in a way that mimics, in part, what happens as you fall asleep. Probably for both these reasons, many people report that they fall asleep more easily after a hot bath.

Sleeping environment also can affect your sleep. Clear your bedroom of any potential sleep distractions, such as noises, bright lights, a television, or computer. Having a comfortable mattress and pillow can help promote a good night's sleep. You also sleep better if the temperature in your bedroom is kept on the cool side. For more ideas on improving your sleep, check out the "Tips for Getting a Good Night's Sleep" on page 30.

Tips for Getting a
Good Night's Sleep

- **Stick to a sleep schedule.** Go to bed and wake up the same time each day. As creatures of habit, people have a hard time adjusting to altered sleep patterns. Sleeping later on weekends won't fully make up for the lack of sleep during the week and will make it harder to wake up early on Monday morning.

- **Exercise is great but not too late in the day.** Try to exercise at least 30 minutes on most days but not later than 5 or 6 hours before your bedtime.

- **Avoid caffeine and nicotine.** Coffee, colas, certain teas, and chocolate contain the stimulant caffeine, and its effects can take as long as 8 hours to wear off fully. Therefore, a cup of coffee in the late afternoon can make it hard for you to fall asleep at night. Nicotine is also a stimulant, often causing smokers to sleep only very lightly. In addition, smokers often wake up too early in the morning because of nicotine withdrawal.

- **Avoid alcoholic drinks before bed.** You may think having an alcoholic "nightcap" will help you sleep, but alcohol robs you of deep sleep and REM sleep, keeping you in the lighter stages of sleep. You also tend to wake up in the middle of the night when the effects of the alcohol have worn off.

- **Avoid large meals and beverages late at night.** A light snack is okay, but a large meal can cause indigestion that interferes with sleep. Drinking too many fluids at night can cause frequent awakenings to urinate.

- **If possible, avoid medicines that delay or disrupt your sleep.** Some commonly prescribed heart, blood pressure, or asthma medications, as well as some over-the-counter and

Good Night's Sleep

herbal remedies for coughs, colds, or allergies, can disrupt sleep patterns. If you have trouble sleeping, talk to your doctor or pharmacist to see if any drugs you're taking might be contributing to your insomnia.

- **Don't take naps after 3 p.m.** Naps can help make up for lost sleep, but late afternoon naps can make it harder to fall asleep at night.

- **Relax before bed.** Don't overschedule your day so that no time is left for unwinding. A relaxing activity, such as reading or listening to music, should be part of your bedtime ritual.

- **Take a hot bath before bed.** The drop in body temperature after getting out of the bath may help you feel sleepy, and the bath can help you relax and slow down so you're more ready to sleep.

- **Have a good sleeping environment.** Get rid of anything that might distract you from sleep, such as noises, bright lights, an uncomfortable bed, or warm temperatures. You sleep better if the temperature in your bedroom is kept on the cool side. A TV or computer in the bedroom can be a distraction and deprive you of needed sleep. Having a comfortable mattress and pillow can help promote a good night's sleep.

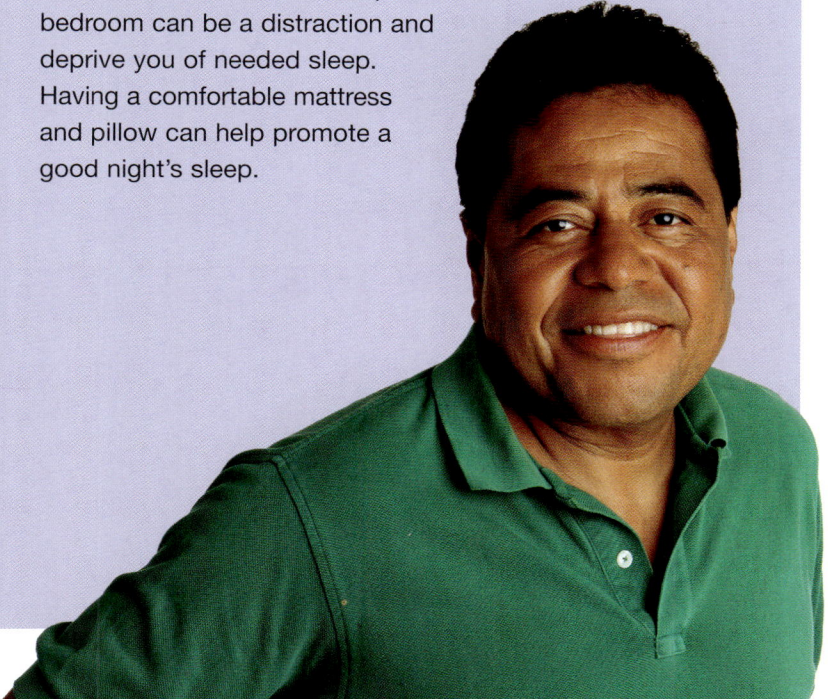

Tips for Getting a
Good Night's Sleep (continued)

- **Have the right sunlight exposure.** Daylight is key to regulating daily sleep patterns. Try to get outside in natural sunlight for at least 30 minutes each day. If possible, wake up with the sun or use very bright lights in the morning. Sleep experts recommend that, if you have problems falling asleep, you should get an hour of exposure to morning sunlight.

- **Don't lie in bed awake.** If you find yourself still awake after staying in bed for more than 20 minutes, get up and do some relaxing activity until you feel sleepy. The anxiety of not being able to sleep can make it harder to fall asleep.

- **See a doctor if you continue to have trouble sleeping.** If you consistently find yourself feeling tired or not well rested during the day despite spending enough time in bed at night, you may have a sleep disorder. Your family doctor or a sleep specialist should be able to help you.

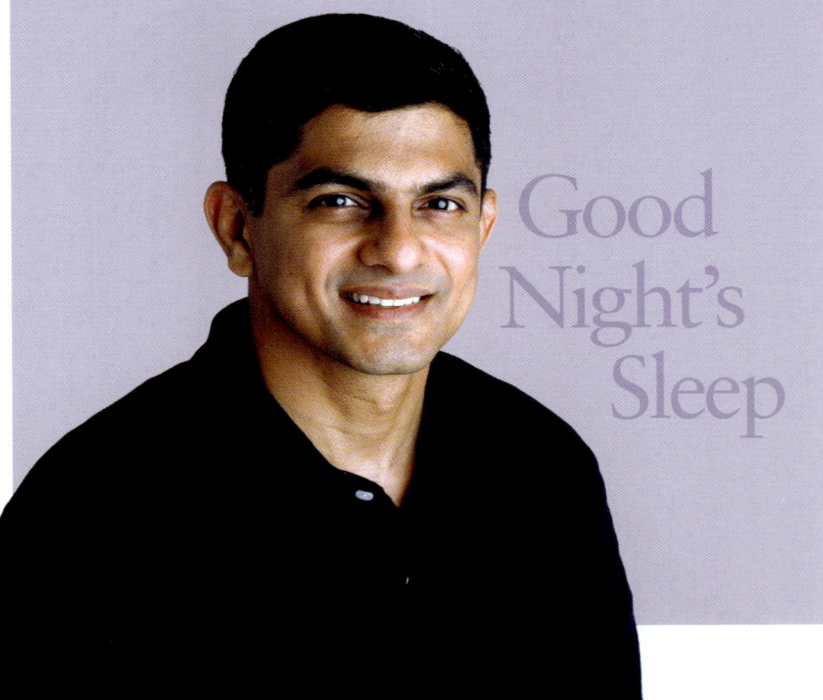

Good
Night's
Sleep

Is Snoring a Problem?

Long the material for jokes, snoring is generally accepted as common and annoying in adults but as nothing to worry about. However, snoring is no laughing matter. Frequent, loud snoring is often a sign of sleep apnea and may increase your risk of developing cardiovascular disease and diabetes, as well as lead to daytime sleepiness and impaired performance.

Snoring is caused by a narrowing or partial blockage of your airways at the back of the mouth and upper throat. This obstruction results in increased air turbulence when breathing in, causing the soft tissues in your throat to vibrate. The end result is a noisy snore that can disrupt the sleep of your bed partner. This narrowing of the airways is typically caused by the soft palate, tongue, and throat relaxing while you sleep, but allergies or sinus problems can also contribute to a narrowing of the airways, as can being overweight and having extra soft tissue around your upper airways.

The larger the tissues in your soft palate, the more likely you are to snore while sleeping. Alcohol or sedatives taken shortly before sleep also promote snoring. These drugs cause greater relaxation of the tissues in your throat and mouth. Surveys reveal that about one-half of all adults snore, and 50 percent of these adults do so loudly and frequently. African Americans, Asians, and Hispanics are more likely to snore loudly and frequently compared to Caucasians, and snoring problems increase with age.

Not everyone who snores has sleep apnea, but people who have sleep apnea typically do snore loudly and frequently. Sleep apnea is a serious sleep disorder, and its hallmark is loud, frequent snoring linked to intermittent brief pauses in breathing while sleeping. (See "Sleep Apnea" on page 40.) Even if you don't experience these breathing pauses, snoring can still be a problem for you as well as for your bed partner. The increased breathing effort associated with snoring can impair your sleep quality and lead to many of the same health consequences as sleep apnea.

One study found that older adults who did not have sleep apnea, but who snored 6–7 nights a week, were more than twice as likely to report being excessively sleepy during the day than those who never snored. The more people snored, the more daytime fatigue they reported. That sleepiness may help explain why snorers are more likely to be in car crashes than people who do not snore. Loud snoring can also disrupt the sleep of bed partners and strain marital relations, especially if snoring causes the spouses to sleep in separate bedrooms.

Snoring also increases the risk of developing diabetes and heart disease. One study found that women who snored regularly were twice as likely as those who did not snore to develop diabetes, even if they were not overweight—another risk factor for diabetes. Other studies suggest persistent snoring may raise the lifetime risk of developing high blood pressure, heart failure, and stroke.

About one-third of all pregnant women begin snoring for the first time during their second trimester. If you are snoring while pregnant, let your doctor know. Snoring in pregnancy can be associated with high blood pressure and can have a negative effect on your baby's growth and development. Your doctor will routinely keep a close eye on your blood pressure throughout your pregnancy and can let you know if any additional evaluations for the snoring might be useful. In most cases, the snoring and any related high blood pressure will subside shortly after delivery.

Snoring can also be a problem in children. As many as 10–15 percent of young children, who typically have enlarged adenoids and tonsils, snore on a regular basis. Several studies show that children who snore (with or without sleep apnea) are more likely than those who do not snore to score lower on tests that measure intelligence, memory, and ability to maintain attention. These children also have more problematic behavior, including hyperactivity. The end result is that children who snore do not perform in school as well as those who do not snore. Strikingly, snoring was linked to a greater drop in IQ than that seen in children who had elevated levels of lead in their blood. Although the behavior of children improves after they stop snoring, studies suggest they may continue to get poorer grades in school, perhaps because of lasting effects on the brain linked to the snoring. You should have your child evaluated by your doctor if the child snores loudly and frequently—three to four times a week—especially if brief pauses in breathing while asleep are noted and if there are signs of hyperactivity or daytime sleepiness, inadequate school achievement, or slower than expected development.

Surgery to remove the adenoids and tonsils of children often can cure their snoring and any associated sleep apnea. Such surgery has been linked to a reduction in hyperactivity and improved ability to pay attention, even in children who showed no signs of sleep apnea before surgery.

Snoring in older children and adults may be relieved by less invasive measures, however. These measures include losing weight, refraining from tobacco, sleeping on the side rather than on the back, or elevating the head while sleeping. Treating chronic congestion and refraining from alcohol or sedatives before sleeping can also stop snoring. In some adults, snoring can be relieved by dental appliances that reposition the soft tissues in the mouth. Although numerous over-the-counter nasal strips and sprays claim to relieve snoring, no scientific evidence supports those claims.

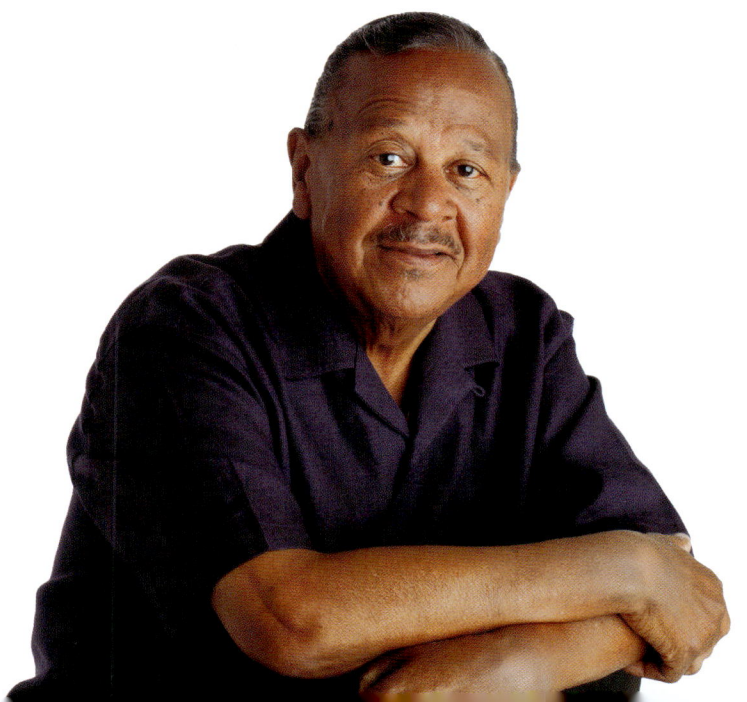

Common Sleep Disorders

A number of sleep disorders can disrupt your sleep quality and leave you with excessive daytime sleepiness, even if enough time was spent in bed to be well rested. (See "Common Signs of a Sleep Disorder" on page 37.) More than 70 sleep disorders affect at least 40 million Americans and account for an estimated $16 billion in medical costs each year, not counting costs due to lost work time and other factors. The four most common sleep disorders are insomnia, obstructive sleep apnea (sleep-disordered breathing), restless legs syndrome (RLS), and narcolepsy. Additional sleep problems include sleep walking, sleep paralysis, night terrors, and other "parasomnias" that cause abnormal arousals.

Insomnia

Insomnia is defined as having trouble falling asleep or staying asleep, or as having unrefreshing sleep despite having ample opportunity to sleep. Life is filled with events that occasionally cause insomnia for a short time. Such temporary insomnia is common and is often brought on by stressful situations such as work, family pressures, or a traumatic event. A National Sleep Foundation poll of adults in the United States found that close to half of the respondents reported temporary insomnia in the nights immediately after the terrorist attacks on September 11, 2001.

Chronic insomnia is defined as having symptoms at least 3 nights per week for more than 1 month. Most cases of chronic insomnia are secondary, which means

Common Signs of a
Sleep Disorder

Look over this list of common signs of a sleep disorders, and talk to your doctor if you have any of them:

- It takes you more than 30 minutes to fall asleep at night.
- You awaken frequently in the night and then have trouble falling back to sleep again.
- You awaken too early in the morning.
- You frequently don't feel well rested despite spending 7–8 hours or more asleep at night.
- You feel sleepy during the day and fall asleep within 5 minutes if you have an opportunity to nap, or you fall asleep at inappropriate times during the day.
- Your bed partner claims you snore loudly, snort, gasp, or make choking sounds while you sleep, or your partner notices your breathing stops for short periods.
- You have creeping, tingling, or crawling feelings in your legs that are relieved by moving or massaging them, especially in the evening and when you try to fall asleep.
- You have vivid, dreamlike experiences while falling asleep or dozing.
- You have episodes of sudden muscle weakness when you are angry, fearful, or when you laugh.
- You feel as though you cannot move when you first wake up.
- Your bed partner notes that your legs or arms jerk often during sleep.
- You regularly need to use stimulants to stay awake during the day.

Also keep in mind that, although children can show some of these same signs of a sleep disorder, they often do not show signs of excessive daytime sleepiness. Instead, they may seem overactive and have difficulty focusing and concentrating. They also may not do their best in school.

Sleep Disorder

they are due to another disorder or medications. Primary chronic insomnia is a distinct sleep disorder; its cause is not yet well understood. About 30–40 percent of adults say they have some symptoms of insomnia within any given year, and about 10–15 percent of adults say they have chronic insomnia. Chronic insomnia becomes more prevalent with age, and women are more likely than men to report having insomnia.

Insomnia often causes problems during the day, such as excessive sleepiness, fatigue, a lack of energy, difficulty concentrating, depressed mood, and irritability. Due to all of these potential consequences, untreated insomnia can impair quality of life as much as, or more than, other chronic medical problems.

Chronic insomnia is often caused by one or more of the following:

- Another disease or mood disorder. The most common causes of insomnia are depression and/or anxiety disorders. Neurological disorders such as Alzheimer's or Parkinson's disease can also have insomnia as a symptom. Chronic insomnia can result from arthritis, asthma, or other medical conditions in which symptoms become more troublesome at night, making it difficult to fall asleep or stay asleep.
- Various prescribed and over-the-counter medications that can disrupt sleep, such as decongestants, certain pain relievers, and steroids.
- Sleep-disrupting behavior such as drinking alcohol, exercising shortly before bedtime, ingesting caffeine late in the day, watching TV or reading while in bed, or irregular sleep schedules due to shift work or other causes.
- Another sleep disorder, such as sleep apnea or restless legs syndrome.

Some people, however, have primary chronic insomnia. This condition is linked to a tendency toward being more "revved up" than normal (hyperarousal). These people may have heightened secretion of certain hormones, higher body temperatures, faster heart rates, and a different pattern of brain waves while they sleep.

Doctors diagnose insomnia based mainly on sleep history, often by reviewing a sleep diary. An overnight sleep recording may be required if another sleep disorder is suspected. Doctors also will try to diagnose and treat any other underlying medical or psychological problems as well as identify behaviors that might be causing the insomnia.

Often, people who have insomnia enter into a vicious cycle—because of having trouble sleeping in previous nights, they become anxious at the slightest sign that they may not be falling asleep right away. That anxiety can make it more difficult for them to fall asleep. The more time they spend in bed not sleeping, and watching the clock, the more their anxiety—and sleeplessness—increases.

To break that cycle of anxiety and negative conditioning, experts recommend going to bed only when you're sleepy. If you can't fall asleep (or fall back to sleep) within 20 minutes, get out of bed and go into another room where you can pursue a relaxing activity until you feel sleepy again. Then return to bed. This reconditioning therapy has been shown to be an effective way to treat insomnia.

Another effective behavioral strategy for some people is relaxation therapy. For example, progressively tense and then relax each of the muscle groups in your body before sleep. Another method is to focus on breathing deeply. Relaxation therapy can provide a needed slowing down period so that you are indeed sleepy when the desired bedtime arrives.

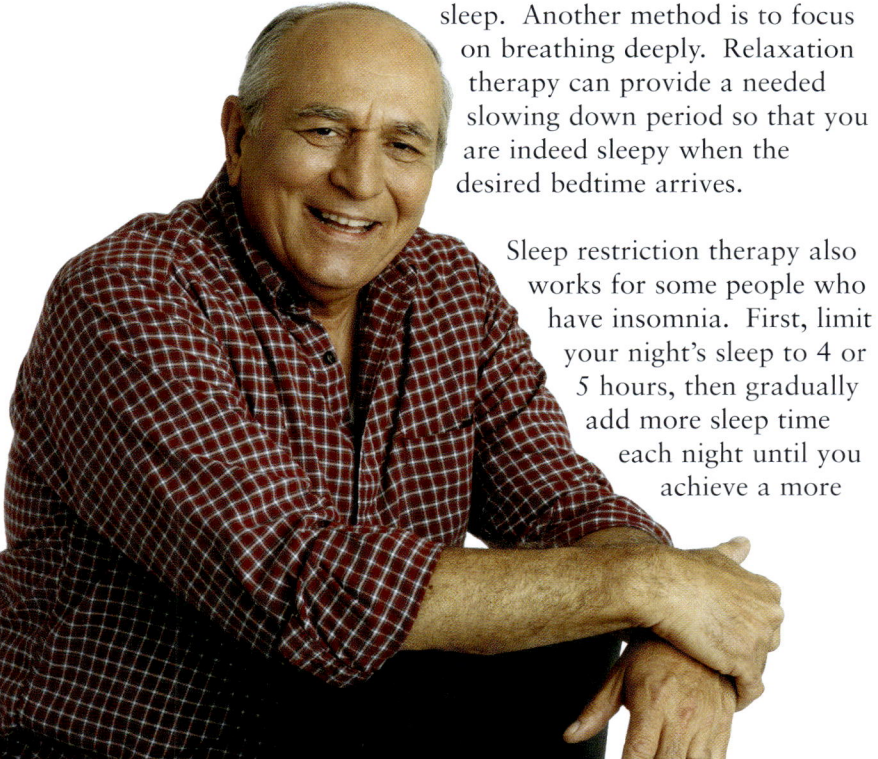

Sleep restriction therapy also works for some people who have insomnia. First, limit your night's sleep to 4 or 5 hours, then gradually add more sleep time each night until you achieve a more normal night's sleep. Daytime naps should be avoided during this sleep restriction therapy because napping may prolong insomnia by making it harder to fall asleep at night. In addition, during sleep restriction therapy, avoid driving a car or operating dangerous machinery until you have obtained adequate nighttime sleep.

All these changes in behavior are part of what is called "cognitive behavioral therapy." Cognitive behavioral therapy also can be used to replace negative thinking related to sleep, such as "I'll never fall asleep without sleeping pills," with more realistic positive thinking. Cognitive behavioral therapy is effective in most people who have chronic insomnia.

Some people who have chronic insomnia that is not corrected by behavioral therapy or treatment of an underlying condition may need a prescription medication. You should talk to a doctor before trying to treat insomnia with alcohol, over-the-counter or prescribed short-acting sedatives, or sedating antihistamines that induce drowsiness. The benefits of these treatments are limited, and they have risks. Some may help you fall asleep but leave you feeling unrefreshed in the morning. Others have longer-lasting effects and leave you feeling still tired and groggy in the morning. Some also may lose their effectiveness over time. Doctors may prescribe sedating antidepressants for insomnia, but the effectiveness of these medicines in people who do not have depression is not established, and there are significant side effects.

To treat their insomnia, some people pursue "natural" remedies, such as melatonin supplements or valerian teas or extracts. These remedies are available over the counter. There is little evidence that melatonin can help relieve insomnia. Studies with valerian have also been inconclusive, and the actual dose and purity of various supplements, extracts, or teas that contain valerian may vary from product to product. In addition, because melatonin, valerian, and other natural remedies are not regulated by the Food and Drug Administration, their safety is not scrutinized.

Sleep Apnea

In people who have sleep apnea (also referred to as sleep-disordered breathing), breathing briefly stops or becomes very shallow during sleep. This change is caused by intermittent blocking of the upper airway, usually when the soft tissue in the rear of the throat

ANNE COLLINS

"I have sleep apnea. In the past, I used to arrange my schedule around whether I've had enough sleep. Now I don't worry about that. Starting on continuous positive airway pressure and medication have changed my life—now I'm excited to wake up and face each day after a night of restful sleep."

collapses and partially or completely closes the airway. Each breathing stop typically lasts 10–20 seconds or more and may occur 20–30 times or more each sleeping hour.

If you have sleep apnea, not enough air can flow into your lungs through the mouth and nose during sleep, even though breathing efforts continue. When this happens, the amount of oxygen in your blood decreases. Your brain responds by awakening you enough to tighten the upper airway muscles and open your windpipe. Normal breaths then start again, often with a loud snort or choking sound. Although people who have sleep apnea typically snore loudly and frequently, not everyone who snores has sleep apnea. (See "Is Snoring a Problem?" on page 33.)

Because people who have sleep apnea frequently arouse from deeper sleep stages to lighter sleep during the night, they rarely spend enough time in deep, restorative stages of sleep. They are therefore often excessively sleepy during the day. Such sleepiness is thought to lead to mood and behavior problems, including depression, and such sleepiness more than triples the risk of being in a traffic or work-related accident.

The many brief drops in blood-oxygen levels can be associated with morning headaches and decreased ability to concentrate, think properly, learn, and remember. In sleep apnea, the combination of the intermittent oxygen drops and reduced sleep quality triggers the release of stress hormones. These hormones in turn raise your blood pressure and heart rate and boost the risk of heart attack, stroke, irregular heart beats, and congestive heart failure. In addition, untreated sleep apnea can lead to altered energy metabolism that increases the risk for developing obesity and diabetes.

Anyone can have sleep apnea. It is estimated that at least 12–18 million American adults have sleep apnea, making it as common as asthma. More than one-half of the people who have sleep apnea are overweight. Sleep apnea is more common in men. More than 1 in 25 middle-aged men and 1 in 50 middle-aged women have sleep apnea along with excessive daytime sleepiness. About 3 percent of children and 10 percent or more of people over age 65 have sleep apnea. This condition occurs more frequently in African Americans, Asians, Native Americans, and Hispanics than in Caucasians.

More than one-half of all people who have sleep apnea are not diagnosed. People who have sleep apnea generally are not aware that their breathing stops in the night. They just notice that they don't feel well rested when they wake up and are sleepy throughout the day. Their bed partners are likely to notice, however, that they snore loudly and frequently and that they often stop breathing briefly while sleeping. Doctors suspect sleep apnea if these symptoms are present, but the diagnosis must be confirmed with overnight sleep monitoring. (See "How Are Sleep Disorders Diagnosed?" on page 44.) This monitoring will reveal pauses in breathing, frequent sleep arousals, and intermittent drops in levels of oxygen in the blood.

Like adults who have sleep apnea, children who have this disorder usually snore loudly, snort or gasp, and have brief stops in breathing while sleeping. Small children often have enlarged tonsils and adenoids that increase their risk for sleep apnea. But doctors may not suspect sleep apnea in children because, instead of showing the typical signs of sleepiness during the day, these children often become agitated and may be considered hyperactive. The effects of sleep apnea in children may include diminished school performance and difficult, aggressive behavior.

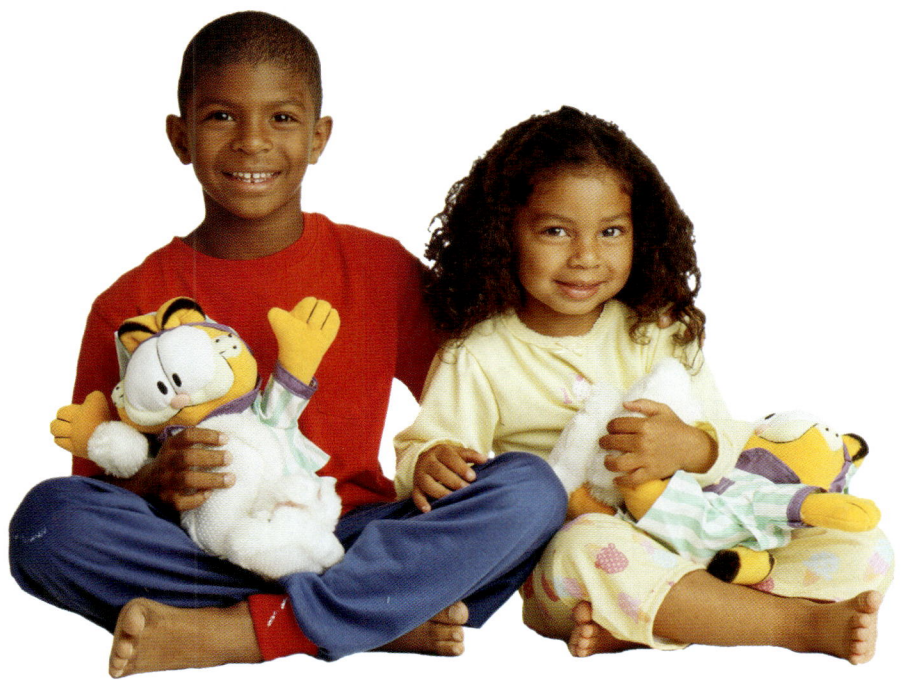

How Are
Sleep Disorders Diagnosed?

Depending on what your symptoms are, your doctor will gather various kinds of information and consider several possible tests when trying to decide if you have a sleep disorder:

- **Sleep history and sleep log.** Your doctor will ask you how many hours you sleep each night, how often you waken during the night and for how long, how long it takes you to fall asleep, how well rested you feel upon awakening, and how sleepy you feel during the day. Your doctor may ask you to keep a sleep diary for a few weeks. (See "Sample Sleep Diary" on page 56.) Your doctor may also ask you if you have any symptoms of sleep apnea or restless legs syndrome, such as loud snoring, snorting or gasping, morning headaches, tingling or unpleasant sensations in the limbs that are relieved by moving them, and jerking of the limbs during sleep. Your sleeping partner may be asked if you have some of these symptoms, as you may not be aware of them yourself.

- **Sleep recording in a sleep lab (polysomnogram).** A sleep recording refers to a polysomnogram (poly-SOM-no-gram) or PSG test that is usually done in a sleep center or sleep laboratory. You will likely stay overnight in the sleep center with electrodes and other monitors placed on your scalp, face, chest, limbs, and finger. While you sleep, these devices measure your brain activity, eye movements, muscle activity, heart rate and rhythm, blood pressure, and how much air moves in and out of your lungs. This test also checks the amount of oxygen in your blood. A PSG test is painless. In certain circumstances, the PSG can be done at home. A home monitor can be used to record heart rate, how air moves in and out of your lungs, the amount of oxygen in your blood, and your breathing effort.

- **Multiple Sleep Latency Test (MSLT).** Particularly useful for diagnosing narcolepsy, this test measures how sleepy you are during the day. In this test, typically done after an overnight sleep recording (PSG), monitoring devices for sleep stage are placed on your scalp and face. You are asked to nap four or five times for 20 minutes every 2 hours during times in which you would normally be awake. Technicians note how quickly you fall asleep and how long it takes you to reach various stages of sleep, especially REM sleep, during your naps. Normal individuals either do not fall asleep during these short designated nap times or take a long time to fall asleep. People who fall asleep in less than 5 minutes are likely to require treatment for a sleep disorder, as are those who quickly develop REM sleep during their naps.

It is important to have a sleep medicine specialist interpret the results of your sleep monitoring test (PSG) or MSLT. See "How To Find a Sleep Center and Sleep Medicine Specialist" on page 58.

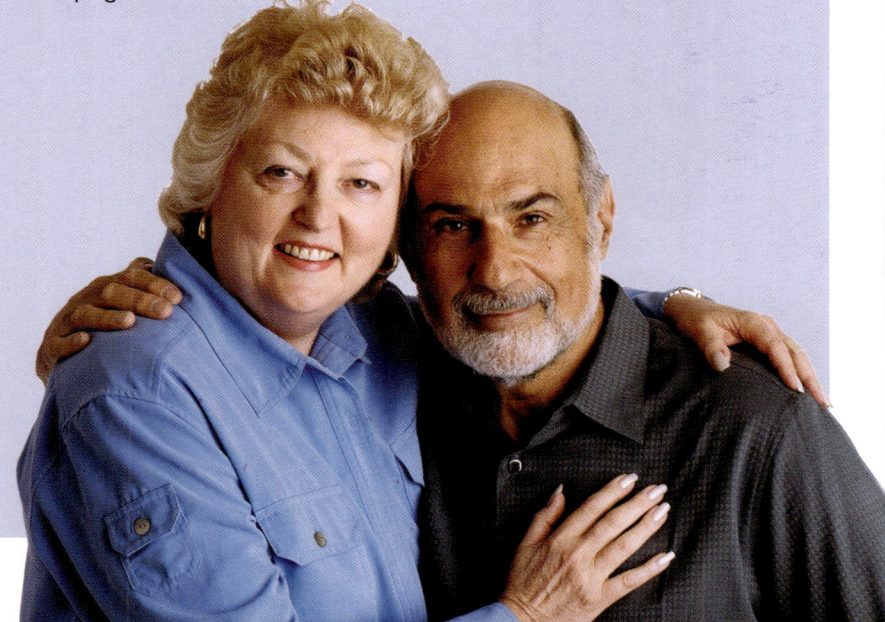

A number of factors can make a person susceptible to sleep apnea. These factors include:

- Throat muscles and tongue that relax more than normal while asleep
- Enlarged tonsils and adenoids
- Being overweight—the excess fat tissue around your neck makes it harder to keep the throat area open
- Head and neck shape that creates a somewhat smaller airway size in the mouth and throat area
- Congestion, due to allergies, that can also narrow the airway
- Family history of sleep apnea

If your doctor suspects that you have sleep apnea, you may be referred to a sleep specialist. Some of the ways to help diagnose sleep apnea include:

- A medical history that includes asking you and your family questions about how you sleep and how you function during the day.
- Checking your mouth, nose, and throat for extra or large tissues—for example tonsils, uvula (the tissue that hangs from the middle of the back of the mouth), and soft palate (roof of your mouth in the back of your throat).
- An overnight recording of what happens with your breathing during sleep (polysomnogram, or PSG).

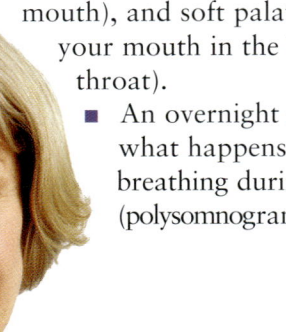

- A Multiple Sleep Latency Test (MSLT), usually done in a sleep center, is used to see how quickly you fall asleep at times when you would normally be awake. Falling asleep in only a few minutes usually means that you are very sleepy during the day. Being very sleepy during the day can be a sign of sleep apnea.

Once all the tests are completed, the sleep medicine specialist will review the results and work with you and your family to develop a treatment plan. Changes in daily activities or habits may help reduce your symptoms:

- **Sleep on your side instead of on your back.** Sleeping on your side will help reduce the amount of upper airway collapse during sleep.
- **Avoid alcohol, smoking, sleeping pills, herbal supplements, and any other medications that make you sleepy.** They make it harder for your airway to stay open while you sleep, and sedatives can make the breathing pauses longer and more severe. Tobacco smoke irritates the airways and can help trigger the intermittent collapse of the upper airway.
- **Lose weight if you are overweight.** Even a little weight loss can sometimes improve symptoms.

These changes may be all that are needed to treat *mild sleep apnea*. However, if you have *moderate or severe sleep apnea*, you will need additional, more direct treatment approaches.

Continuous Positive Airway Pressure (CPAP) is the most effective treatment for sleep apnea in adults. CPAP delivers air into your airway through a specially designed nasal mask attached to a machine that acts as a pump. The mask does not breathe for you; the flow of air creates enough increased pressure to keep the airways in your nose and mouth more open while you sleep. The air pressure is adjusted so that it is just enough to stop your airways from briefly becoming too small during sleep. The pressure is constant and continuous. Sleep apnea will return if CPAP is stopped or if it is used incorrectly.

People who have severe sleep apnea symptoms generally feel much better once they begin treatment with CPAP. CPAP treatment can cause side effects in some people. Possible side effects include dry or stuffy nose, irritation of the skin on the face, bloating of the stomach, sore eyes, or headaches. If you have trouble with CPAP side effects,

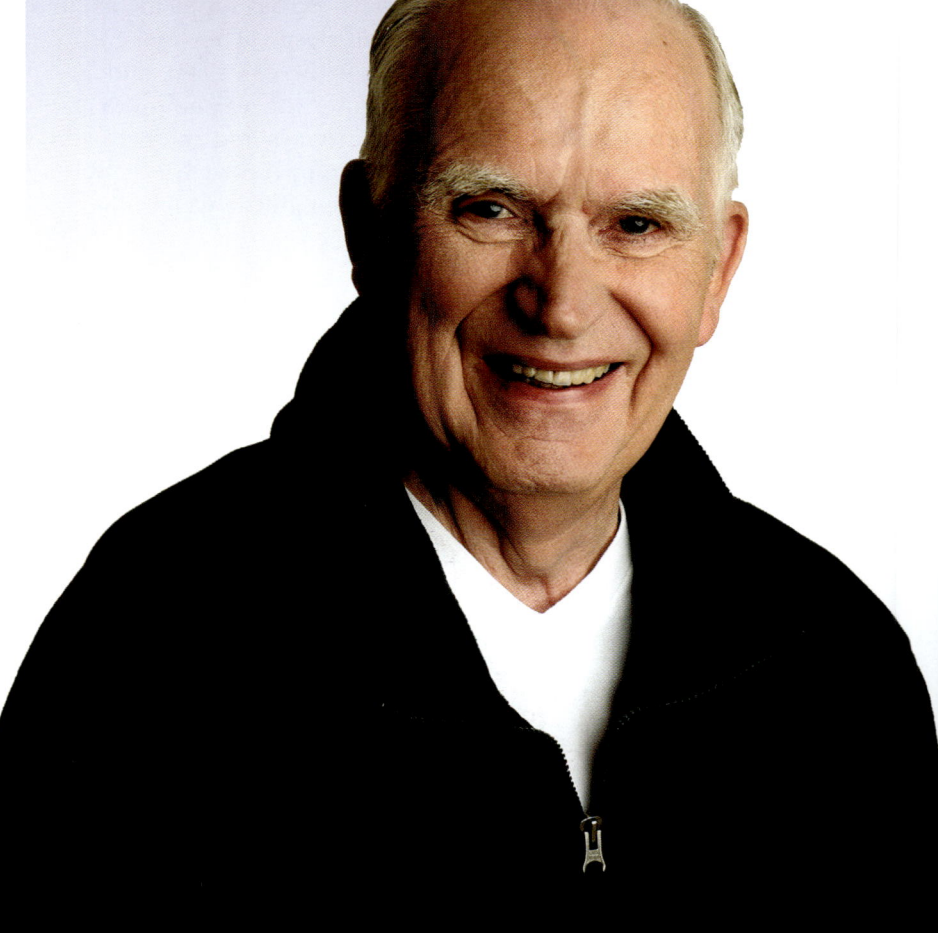

"With restless legs syndrome, there is no 'magic bullet,' no cure. It took a while to find the correct combination of medications for me. From time to time, my medications have to be adjusted, but my symptoms are well controlled."

work with your sleep medicine specialist and support staff. Together, you can do things to reduce or eliminate these problems.

Currently, no medications cure sleep apnea. However, the prescription drug modafinil may help relieve the excessive sleepiness that sometimes persists even with CPAP treatment of sleep apnea.

Another treatment approach that may help some people is the use of a mouthpiece (oral or dental appliance). If you have mild sleep apnea or do not have sleep apnea but snore very loudly, your doctor or dentist may also recommend this. A custom-fitted plastic mouthpiece will be made by a dentist or an orthodontist—a specialist in correcting teeth or jaw problems. The mouthpiece will adjust your lower jaw and tongue to help keep the airway in your throat more open while you are sleeping. Air can then flow more easily into your lungs because there is less resistance to breathing. Following up with the dentist or orthodontist is important to correct any side effects and to be sure that your mouthpiece continues to fit properly.

Some people who have sleep apnea, depending on the findings of the evaluation by the sleep medicine specialist, may benefit from surgery. Removing tonsils and adenoids that are blocking the airway is done frequently, especially in children. Uvulopalatopharyngoplasty (UPPP) is a surgery for adults that removes the tonsils, uvula (the tissue that hangs from the middle of the back of the roof of the mouth), and part of the soft palate (roof of the mouth in the back of the throat). Tracheostomy is a surgery used rarely and only in severe sleep apnea when no other treatments have been successful. A small hole is made in the windpipe, and a tube is inserted. Air will flow through the tube and into the lungs, bypassing the obstruction in the upper airway.

Restless Legs Syndrome (RLS)
Restless legs syndrome (RLS) causes an unpleasant prickling or tingling in the legs, especially in the calves, that is relieved by moving or massaging them. This sensation creates a need to stretch or move the legs to get rid of these uncomfortable or painful feelings. As a result, a person may have difficulty falling asleep and staying asleep. One or both legs may be affected. In some people, the sensations are also felt in the arms. These sensations can also occur with lying down or sitting for prolonged periods of time, such as while at a desk, riding in a car, or watching a movie.

Many people who have RLS also have brief limb movements during sleep, often with abrupt onset, occurring every 5–90 seconds. This condition, known as periodic limb movements in sleep (PLMS), can repeatedly awaken people who have RLS and reduce their total sleep time. Some people have PLMS but have no abnormal sensations in their legs while awake.

RLS affects 5–15 percent of Americans, and its prevalence increases with age. RLS occurs more often in women than men. One study found that RLS accounted for one-third of the insomnia seen in patients older than age 60. Children also can have RLS. This condition can be difficult to diagnose in children, and it often is confused with hyperactivity or "growing pains."

RLS is often inherited. Pregnancy, kidney failure, and anemia related to iron or vitamin deficiency can trigger or worsen RLS symptoms. Researchers suspect that these conditions cause insufficient iron that results in a lack of dopamine. The brain uses dopamine to control limb movements. Doctors usually can diagnose RLS by patients' symptoms and a telltale worsening of symptoms at night or while at rest. Some doctors may order a blood test for iron, although many people who have RLS have normal levels of iron in their blood but abnormal levels in the fluid that bathes their brain. Doctors may also ask people who have RLS to spend a night in a sleep lab where they are monitored to rule out other sleep disorders and to document the excessive limb movements.

RLS is a treatable but not curable condition. Dramatic improvements are seen quickly when patients are given dopamine-like drugs. Alternatively, people who have milder cases may be treated successfully with sedatives or by behavioral strategies. These strategies include stretching, taking a hot bath, or massaging the legs before bedtime. Avoiding caffeinated beverages can also help reduce symptoms. If iron or vitamin deficiency underlies RLS, symptoms may improve with prescribed iron, vitamin B12, or folate supplements. Some people may require anticonvulsant medications to stem the creeping and crawling sensations in their limbs. Others who have severe symptoms may need to be treated with pain relievers, such as codeine or morphine, or a combination of drug treatments.

Narcolepsy

Narcolepsy's main symptom is excessive and overwhelming daytime sleepiness, even after adequate nighttime sleep. In addition, night-time sleep may be fragmented by frequent awakenings. People who have narcolepsy often fall asleep at inappropriate times and places. Although television sitcoms occasionally feature these individuals to generate a few laughs, narcolepsy is no laughing matter. People who have narcolepsy experience daytime "sleep attacks" that last from seconds to more than one-half hour, can occur without warning, and may cause injury. These embarrassing sleep spells can also make it difficult to work and to maintain normal personal or social relationships.

With narcolepsy, the usually sharp distinctions between being asleep and awake are blurred. Also, people who have narcolepsy tend to fall directly into dream-filled REM sleep, rather than enter REM sleep gradually after passing through the non-REM sleep stages first.

In addition to overwhelming daytime sleepiness, narcolepsy has three other commonly associated symptoms, but these may not occur in all people:

- **Sudden muscle weakness (cataplexy).** This weakness is similar to the paralysis that normally occurs during REM sleep, but it lasts a few seconds to minutes while an individual is awake. Cataplexy tends to be triggered by sudden emotional reactions, such as anger, surprise, fear, or laughter. The weakness may show up as limpness at the neck, buckling of the knees, or sagging facial muscles affecting speech, or it may cause a complete body collapse.
- **Sleep paralysis.** People who have narcolepsy may experience a temporary inability to talk or move when falling asleep or waking up, as if they were glued to their beds.
- **Vivid (hypnogogic) dreams.** These dreams tend to surface when people who have narcolepsy first fall asleep. The dreams are so lifelike that they can be confused with reality.

Experts estimate that as many as 350,000 Americans have narcolepsy, but fewer than 50,000 are diagnosed. The disorder is as widespread as

BOB BALKAM

❝When you have a sleep disorder, you need to discuss your symptoms and progress so your doctor can know when it's necessary to change the course of treatment. Patient support groups are also invaluable sources of information.❞

Parkinson's disease or multiple sclerosis, and more prevalent than cystic fibrosis, but it is less well known. Narcolepsy is often mistaken for depression, epilepsy, or the side effects of medicines.

Narcolepsy can be difficult to diagnose in people who have only the symptom of excessive daytime sleepiness. It is usually diagnosed with the aid of an overnight sleep recording (PSG) and the MSLT. (See "How Are Sleep Disorders Diagnosed?" on page 44.) Both tests reveal signs of narcolepsy—the tendency to fall asleep rapidly and enter REM sleep early, even during brief naps.

Narcolepsy can develop at any age, but the symptoms tend to appear first during adolescence or early adulthood. About 1 of every 10 people who have narcolepsy has a close family member who has the disorder, suggesting that one can inherit a tendency to develop narcolepsy. Studies suggest that a neurotransmitter called hypocretin plays a key role in narcolepsy. Most people who have narcolepsy lack hypocretin, which promotes wakefulness. Scientists believe that an autoimmune reaction, perhaps triggered by disease or brain injury, specifically destroys the hypocretin-generating cells in the brains of people who have narcolepsy.

Eventually, researchers may develop a treatment for narcolepsy that restores hypocretin to normal levels. In the meantime, most people who have narcolepsy find some to all of their symptoms relieved by various drug treatments. For example, central nervous system stimulants can reduce daytime sleepiness. Antidepressants and other drugs that suppress REM sleep can prevent muscle weakness, sleep paralysis, and vivid dreaming. Doctors also usually recommend that people who have narcolepsy take short naps (10–15 minutes) two or three times a day, if possible, to help control excessive daytime sleepiness.

Parasomnias (Abnormal Arousals)

In some people, the walking, talking, and other body functions normally suppressed during sleep emerge during certain sleep stages. Alternatively, the paralysis or vivid images usually experienced during dreaming may persist after awakening. These arousal malfunctions are collectively known as parasomnias and include confusional arousals, sleep talking, sleep walking, night terrors, sleep paralysis, and REM sleep behavior disorder (acting out dreams). Most of these disorders—such as confusional arousals, sleep walking, and night terrors—are more common in children, who tend to outgrow them once they become adults. People who are sleep-deprived also may experience some of these disorders, including sleep walking and sleep paralysis. Sleep paralysis also commonly occurs in people who have narcolepsy. Certain medications or neurological disorders appear to lead to other parasomnias, such as REM sleep behavior disorder, and these parasomnias tend to occur more in elderly people. If you or a family member has persistent episodes of sleep paralysis, sleep walking, or acting out of dreams, talk with your doctor.

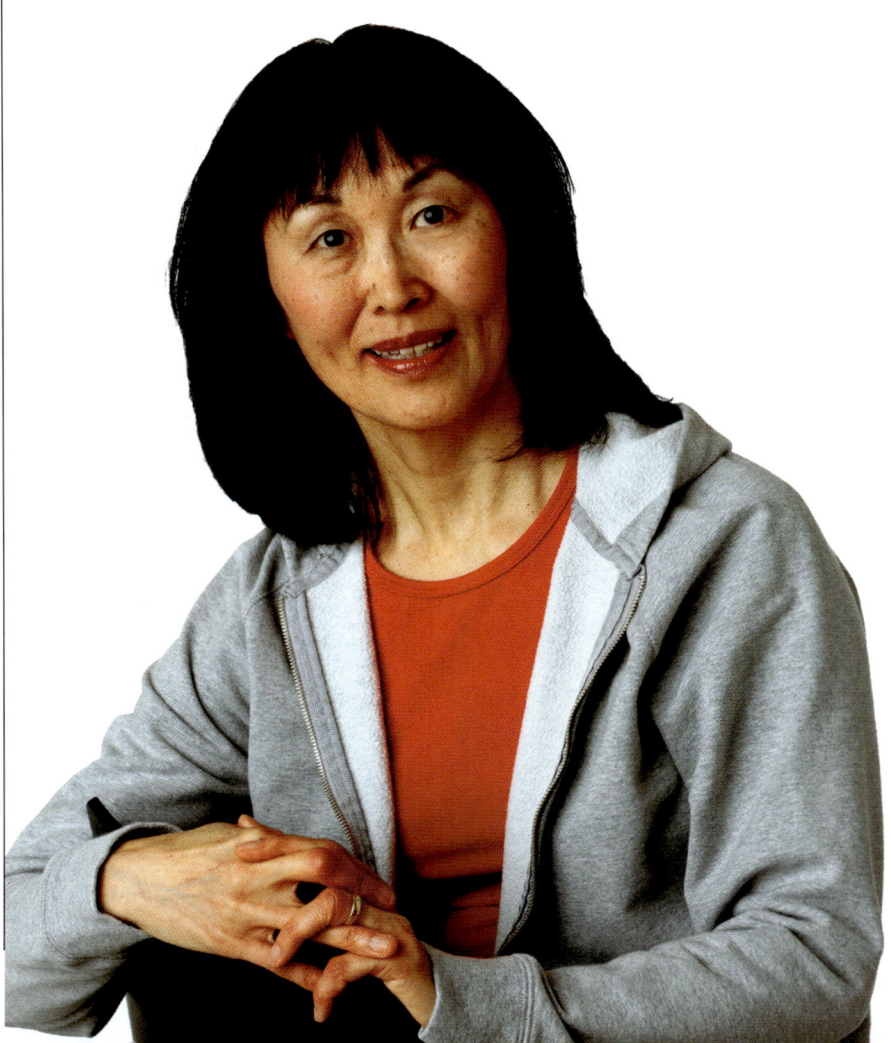

Do You Think You Have a Sleep Disorder?

At various points in our lives, all of us suffer from a lack of sleep that can be remedied by making sure we have the opportunity to get enough sleep. But, if you are spending enough time in bed and still wake up tired or feel very sleepy during the day, you may have a sleep disorder. See "Common Signs of a Sleep Disorder" on page 37.

One of the best ways you can tell if you are getting enough good quality sleep, and whether you have signs of a sleep disorder, is by keeping a sleep diary. Use the "Sample Sleep Diary" on page 56 to record the quality and quantity of your sleep; your use of medications, alcohol, and caffeinated beverages; your exercise patterns; and how sleepy you feel during the day. After a week or so, look over this information to see how many hours of sleep or nighttime awakenings the night before are linked to your being tired the next day. This information will give you a sense of how much uninterrupted sleep you need to avoid daytime sleepiness. You can also use the diary to see some of the patterns or practices that may keep you from getting a good night's sleep.

You may have a sleep disorder and should see your doctor if your sleep diary reveals any of the following:

- You consistently take more than 30 minutes each night to fall asleep.
- You consistently awaken more than a few times or for long periods of time each night.
- You take frequent naps.
- You often feel sleepy during the day—especially if you fall asleep at inappropriate times during the day.

Sample Sleep Diary

Name	Example			
Today's date	**Monday 4/10/05**			
Complete in the Morning — Time I went to bed last night	11 p.m.			
Time I woke up this morning	7 a.m.			
No. of hours slept last night	8			
Number of awakenings and total time awake last night	5 times 2 hours			
How long I took to fall asleep last night	30 mins.			
Medications taken last night	None			
How awake did I feel when I got up this morning: 1—Wide awake 2—Awake but a little tired 3—Sleepy	2			
Complete in the Evening — Number of caffeinated drinks (coffee, tea, soda) and time when I had them today	1 drink at 8 p.m.			
Number of alcoholic drinks (beer, wine, liquor) and time when I had them today	2 drinks 9 p.m.			
Nap times and lengths today	3:30 p.m. 45 mins.			
Exercise times and lengths today	None			
How sleepy did I feel during the day today: 1—So sleepy had to struggle to stay awake during much of the day 2—Somewhat tired 3—Fairly alert 4—Wide awake	1			

How To Find a Sleep Center and Sleep Medicine Specialist

If your doctor refers you to a sleep center or sleep specialist, make sure that center or specialist is qualified to diagnose and treat your sleep problem. To find sleep centers accredited by the American Academy of Sleep Medicine, go to http://www.aasmnet.org and click on "Find a Sleep Center," or call 708–492–0930. To find sleep specialists certified by the American Board of Sleep Medicine, go to http://www.absm.org and click on "Diplomates of the ABSM."

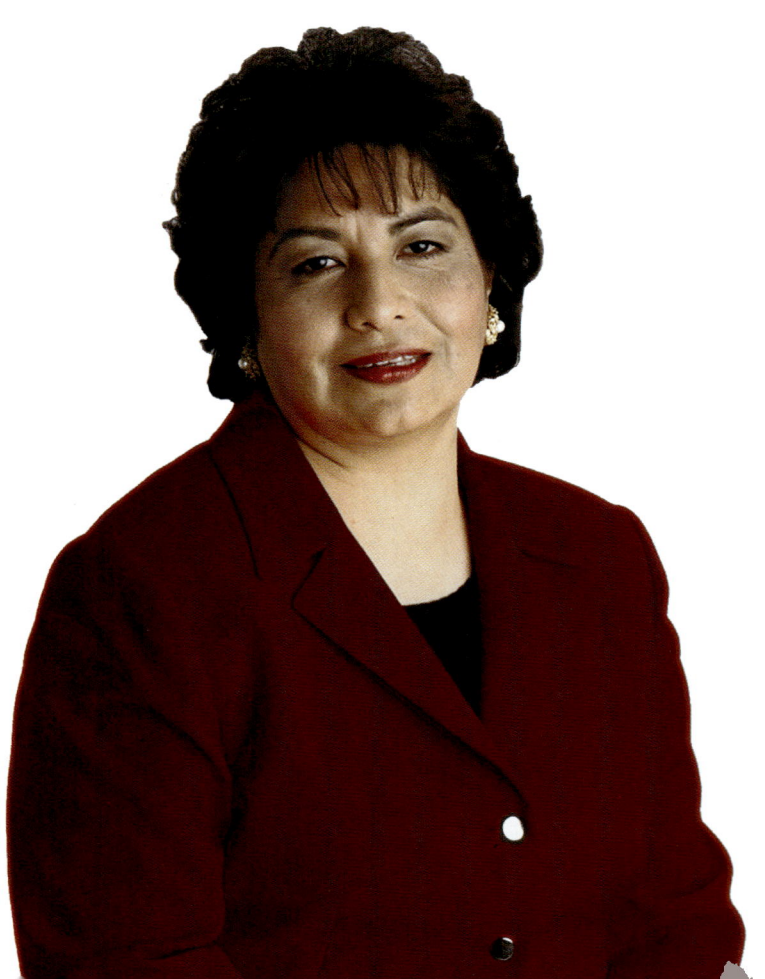

For More Sleep Information

Resources from the National Heart, Lung, and Blood Institute (NHLBI)
National Center on Sleep Disorders Research
National Heart, Lung, and Blood Institute
National Institutes of Health
6705 Rockledge Drive
Suite 6022
Bethesda, MD 20892–7993
Telephone: 301–435–0199
Fax: 301–480–3451
E-mail: ncsdr@nih.gov
Web site: http://www.nhlbi.nih.gov/sleep

NHLBI Health Information Center
P.O. Box 30105
Bethesda, MD 20824–0105
Telephone: 301–592–8573
TTY: 240–629–3255
Fax: 301–592–8563
E-mail: nhlbiinfo@nhlbi.nih.gov
Web site: http://www.nhlbi.nih.gov

Garfield Star Sleeper Web site (for children, parents, and teachers)
http://starsleep.nhlbi.nih.gov

NIH Office of Science Education Web site (for high school supplemental curriculum: Sleep, Sleep Disorders, and Biological Rhythms)
http://science.education.nih.gov

Resources from Other Sleep Organizations
American Academy of Sleep Medicine (AASM)
One Westbrook Corporate Center, Suite 920
Westchester, IL 60154
Telephone: 708–492–0930
Fax: 708–492–0943
Web site: http://www.aasmnet.org

American Insomnia Association
(same address/phone as AASM)
E-mail: rmoney@aasmnet.org
Web site: http://www.americaninsomniaassociation.org

American Sleep Apnea Association
1424 K Street, NW
Suite 302
Washington, DC 20005
Telephone: 202–293–3650
Fax: 202–293–3656
Web site: http://www.sleepapnea.org

Narcolepsy Network, Inc.
P.O. Box 294
Pleasantville, NY 10570
Telephone: 401–667–2523
Fax: 401–633–6567
E-mail: narnet@narcolepsynetwork.org
Web site: http://www.narcolepsynetwork.org

National Sleep Foundation
1522 K Street, NW
Suite 500
Washington, DC 20005
Telephone: 202–347–3471
Fax: 202–347–3472
E-mail: nsf@sleepfoundation.org
Web site: http://www.sleepfoundation.org

Restless Legs Syndrome Foundation
819 Second Street, SW
Rochester, MN 55902–2985
Telephone: 507–287–6465
Fax: 507–287–6312
E-mail: rlsfoundation@rls.org
Web site: http://www.rls.org